AF714960

6 Frontiers in European Radiology

Editors-in-Chief

A. L. Baert · E. Boijsen
W. A. Fuchs · F. H. W. Heuck

Coordinating Editor of this Volume: F. H. W. Heuck

Editorial Board

P. Bodart · G. Breitling · L. Dalla-Palma · W. Dihlmann
G. du Boulay · P. Edholm · C. Fauré · H. Frommhold
W. Frommhold · T. Greitz · V. Hegedüs · H. Kaufmann
E. Koivisto · L. Kreel · M. Laval-Jeantet · A. Lunderquist
I. Obrez · F. Pinet · H. Pokieser · J. Remy · P. Rossi
T. Sherwood · A. Wackenheim · F. Weill

Springer-Verlag
Berlin Heidelberg New York
London Paris Tokyo

Professor Dr. Albert L. Baert
Universitaire Ziekenhuizen, Department of Diagnostic Radiology,
Kapucijnenvoer 33, B-3000 Leuven

Professor Dr. Erik Boijsen
University Hospital, Department of Diagnostic Radiology, S-22185 Lund

Professor Dr. Walter A. Fuchs
Inselspital Bern, Institut für Diagnostische Radiologie der Universität,
CH-3010 Bern

Professor Dr. Friedrich H.W. Heuck
Hermann-Kurz-Straße 5, D-7000 Stuttgart 1

With 43 Figures (in 100 Separate Illustrations) and 15 Tables

ISBN-13:978-3-642-74235-4 e-ISBN-13:978-3-642-74233-0
DOI: 10.1007/978-3-642-74233-0

This work is subject to copyright. All rights are reserved, whether the whole or part of the material is concerned, specifically the rights of translation, reprinting, re-use of illustrations, recitation, broadcasting, reproduction on microfilms or in other ways, and storage in data banks. Duplication of this publication or parts thereof is only permitted under the provisions of the German Copyright Law of September 9, 1965, in its version of June 24, 1985, and a copyright fee must always be paid. Violations fall under the prosecution act of the German Copyright Law.

© Springer-Verlag Berlin Heidelberg 1989.
Softcover reprint of the hardcover 1st edition 1989

The use of registered names, trademarks. etc. in this publication does not imply, even in the absence of a specific statement, that such names are exempt from the relevant protective laws and regulations and therefore free for general use.

Product Liability: The publisher can give no guarantee for information about drug dosage and application thereof contained in this book. In every individual case the respective user must check its accuracy by consulting other pharmaceutical literature.

Typesetting: Kutschbach, Berlin

2121/3020-543210 – Printed on acid-free paper

Contents

Magnetic Resonance Imaging of Focal Lesions of Liver and Spleen Using Gradient-Echo Sequences at 1.5 Tesla: A Comparison with Ultrasound and Sequential Computerized Tomography

J. Griebel, C.F. Hess, and B. Kurtz[1]

1 Introduction

Ultrasound (US) and computerized tomography (CT) are two well-established methods for diagnostic imaging of the upper abdomen which demonstrate focal changes of the liver with great sensitivity. However, even with adjunctive use of contrast medium-enhanced sequential CT, the differential diagnosis of liver lesions and the demonstration of circumscribed changes of the spleen are not satisfactory with these methods. Puncture-cytologic or histologic assessment of liver lesions, or splenectomy with subsequent histologic assessment, is therefore frequently necessary to clarify the clinical picture.

Conventional magnetic resonance imaging (MRI) has also failed to reduce this problem appreciably. Especially at high field strengths, the acquisition is furthermore affected by interference from respiratory artifacts (*Wood* and *Henkelman* 1986; *Heiken* et

[1] Radiologische Klinik (Dir.: Prof. Dr. Dr. h.c. mult. Walter Frommhold) der Universität Tübingen, Röntgenweg 11, D-7400 Tübingen, FRG

al. 1985). Various techniques, including respiratory gating and signal averaging, have been developed to reduce these motion artifacts (*Stark* et al. 1986; *Bydder* and *Young* 1985a; *Runge* et al. 1984). Nevertheless, even these methods do not satisfactorily eliminate the pronounced imaging artifacts at high field strengths.

Gradient-echo sequences like FLASH (fast low angle shot), described by *Haase* et al. 1986 and *van der Meulen* et al. 1985, are one solution to this problem. Since they allow measurement times of a few seconds, MRI assessment of the upper abdomen can be performed in suspended respiration.

Whereas this new MRI technique has already been repeatedly applied in individual clinical examples (*Haase* et al. 1986; *van der Meulen* et al. 1985; *Edelman* et al. 1986), few reports are available on how focal changes of liver and spleen are demonstrated with FLASH sequences. The aims of our study, therefore, were the following:

1. To establish the characteristic appearance of important circumscribed liver and spleen lesions on MRI with FLASH sequences
2. To establish suitable measurement parameters for evaluation of liver and spleen
3. To discuss the clinical efficacy of MRI with FLASH sequences in comparison with US and sequential CT

2 Methods

The MR scans were performed with a superconductive magnetic system (Magnetom, Siemens) at 1.5 T using FLASH sequences based on the principle of gradient echo (*Haase* et al. 1986; *van der Meulen* et al. 1985) with flip angles smaller than 90°. The echo delay time was 16 ms (Table 1). Repetition time, matrix size, and number of data acquisitions were selected so that a measurement time of 10 s was not exceeded and the scans could be performed in suspended respiration (in expiration). Axial sections were produced by the single-slice technique. The signal course was analyzed with up to 12 different flip angles in that section in which the relevant structures were most optimally demonstrated.

The US scans were performed with a 3.5-MHz sector scanner (Sonoline SL, Siemens) or a 3.5-MHz curved-array scanner (LSC 7000, Picker). The organs were screened for circumscribed changes in intercostal, transverse, and longitudinal sections. All focal lesions of liver or spleen were documented in two mutually perpendicular planes. In addition, the maximal craniocaudal and mediolateral diameters of the spleen were determined in patients with diagnosed malignant lymphoma.

Table 1. Methods

FLASH sequences	
Flip angle	$< 90°$
Echo delay time	16 ms
Repetition time	80 ms
Matrix	128 × 128
No. of data acquisitions	1
Measurement time per scan	10 s

The sequential CT scans were performed with a whole-body scanner (Somatom DR3, Siemens). Sequential scanning was done in that plain CT or US plane showing the greatest extension of the focal lesion. When CT findings were negative, the height of the lesion was marked on the skin under US control in the same position and respiratory phase. Concurrent with the start of the examination, 50 ml of 60 % water-soluble contrast medium was injected manually into the cubital vein (flow rate ca. 10 ml/s). Scan intervals of 5 s were selected in the first 30 s after injection, then 15 s up to 2 min.

Each patient was examined within a 2-week period by all three imaging methods. The authors evaluated all CT and MR scans as well as US documentation together.

3 Patients

3.1 Normal Group

The demonstration of the normal anatomy and the imaging characteristics were investigated by FLASH sequences in a group of 15 healthy volunteers between 18 and 36 years of age (Table 2).

Table 2. Patients

			no
Healthy volunteers			15
Liver study			30
	Hemangioma	8	
	Echinococcus cyst	1	
	FNH	1	
	Gummata	1	
	Metastasis	8	
	Primary hepatocellular carcinoma	5	
	Lymphatic infiltration	6	
Spleen study			24
	Lymphatic infiltration	18	
	Infarct	3	
	Leukosis	1	
	Sarcoidosis	1	
	Primarily unknown etiology	1	
Total			69

3.2 Focal Liver Lesions

Eight patients with hemangiomas of the liver, one with focal nodular hyperplasia, one with an echinococcus cyst, one with luetic gummata (syphiloma) of the liver, eight with liver metastases (three from breast cancer, three from colon cancer, one from cervical cancer, one from carcinoid tumor), five with hepatocellular carcinoma, and six with lymphomatous involvement of the liver (three non-Hodgkin's lymphoma, three Hodgkin's disease) were examined by US, sequential CT, and MRI (Table 2). The diagnosis of hemangioma was confirmed by sequential CT; arteriography was necessary in only one case. In five patients with liver metastases and two patients with lymphomatous involvement of the liver, the diagnosis was obvious on the basis of the clinical course. All other liver lesions were confirmed by puncture-cytologic or histologic assessment.

3.3 Focal Spleen Lesions

After the initial US examination, sequential CT and FLASH MRI were performed to clarify the spleen findings in 24 patients (Table 2). The selection of CT and MRI was based on US findings: Eighteen patients had histologically confirmed malignant lymphoma (seven Hodgkin's disease, 11 non-Hodgkin's lymphoma). In 10 of these patients, US showed focal changes of the spleen which were caused by lymphatic infiltration, as determined by the course of the disease; the diagnosis was confirmed after splenectomy in three patients. On US the spleen of the remaining eight patients with malignant lymphoma appeared homogeneous; four of these patients had severe splenomegaly (max. diameter 14 cm) and one had lymphatic involvement of the liver. A staging laparatomy was performed at a later date in the other three patients with negative US findings.

In one patient with circumscribed infiltration of Hodgkin's disease, the course of the disease was assessed monthly by all three imaging methods for a period of 6 months.

Six patients with spleen lesions of non-lymphatic origin were also evaluated by sequential CT and MRI: three with suspected fresh splenic infarction (acute pain in left upper abdomen, echo-poor areas on US), one with splenic involvement due to sarcoidosis (multiple echo-poor foci in spleen), one with splenic involvement due to leukemia, and one with circumscribed echo-dense changes in the spleen of primarily unknown etiology (primary disease: atrial fibrillation).

4 Fundamentals of FLASH Sequences

FLASH sequences differ fundamentally from conventional spin-echo or inversion-recovery sequences. The pulse and gradient timing is shown in Fig. 1. In contrast to conventional sequences, FLASH sequences utilize radiofrequency (RF) pulses which result in flip angles smaller than 90° and are based on the principle of gradient echo (*Haase* et al. 1986; *van der Meulen* et al. 1985). Furthermore, the refocusing 180° pulse typical for spin-echo sequences is absent.

FLASH sequences have three parameters: repetition time TR, echo delay time TE, and flip angle. Several important consequences for these parameters can be summarized as follows:

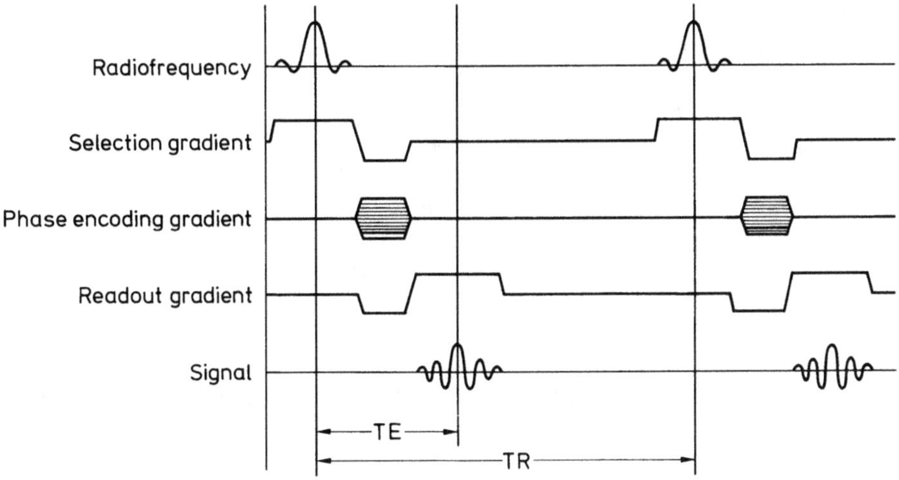

Fig. 1. Pulse and gradient timing for FLASH sequences

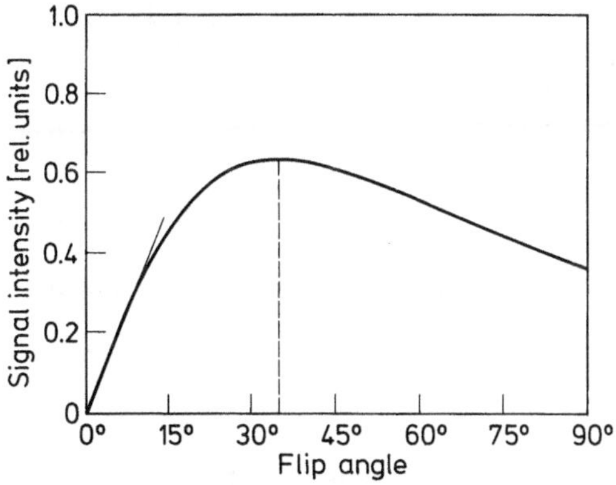

Fig. 2. Theoretical signal course as function of flip angle

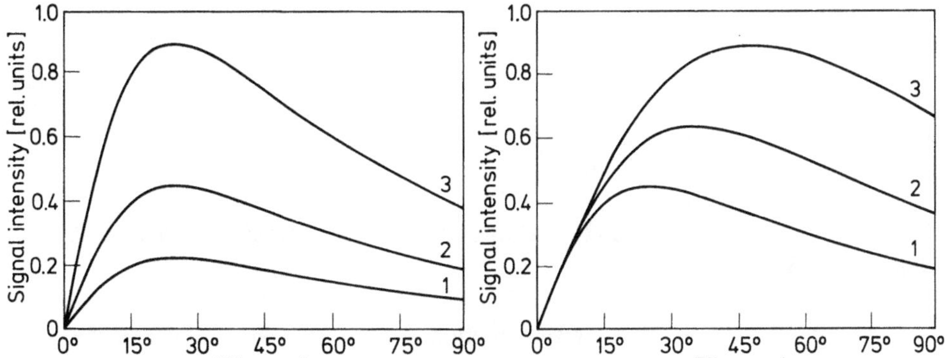

Fig. 3a, b. Theoretical signal course as function of flip angle with variation of tissue parameters. **a** Dependent relation between initial increase and relaxation time T2* or proton density rho; initial increase rises with increasing T2* or rho (1-2-3). **b** Dependent relation between Ernst angle and relaxation time T1; Ernst angle decreases with increasing T1 (3-2-1)

1. Due to the absence of the 180° pulse, TR, and therefore also measurement time, can be drastically shortened (*Haase* et al. 1986; *van der Meulen* et al. 1985). Consequently, the TR selected for diagnostic imaging of the upper abdomen should be as short as possible so that the examination can be done in suspended respiration.
2. As with spin-echo sequences, the signal declines exponentially with increasing TE. Due to the absence of the 180° pulse, however, this decay follows the effective relaxation time T2* rather than relaxation time T2. T2* describes the dephasing of the magnetic nuclear moments under the influence of both the spin-spin relaxation time T2 characteristic for the tissue and the inhomogeneities of the external magnetic field. Since the signal decay of T2* is steeper than that of T2, small values are selected for TE.
3. The variation range for TR und TE is consequently greatly limited; image contrast, therefore, is determined primarily by the selection of the flip angle (*Edelman* et al. 1986; *Griebel* et al. 1987).

The signal course with increasing flip angle, however, differs fundamentally from that with spin-echo or inversion-recovery sequences in that it shows a peak (*Ernst* and *Anderson* 1966) (Fig. 2). The course of the curves is characterized by the initial increase of the peak as well as its position and height (*Klose* et al. 1986; *Griebel* et al. 1987).

The steepness of the initial increase depends on both relaxation time T2* and proton density rho. The equation for the initial increase (m) is

$$m = \text{rho} \cdot \exp(-\text{TE}/\text{T2*}).$$

It rises as T2* or rho increases (Fig. 3a) (*Klose* et al. 1986).

By contrast, the flip angle at which the peak appears, i.e., the Ernst angle, depends solely on T1. The equation for the Ernst angle is

$$\cos(d_{\text{Ernst}}) = \exp(-\text{TR}/\text{T1}).$$

Tissues with long T1 peak at small flip angles, tissues with short T1 at large flip angles (Fig. 3b) (*Ernst* and *Anderson* 1966).

5 Results

5.1 Demonstration of Normal Anatomy and Special Imaging Characteristics Using FLASH Sequences

The structures affected by respiratory motion, e.g., liver, spleen, and kidneys, were imaged without respiratory artifacts in all subjects (Fig. 4a, b).

At large flip angles, fatty tissue, in addition to the vessels, imaged as the most signal-dense structure and therefore contributed essentially to the image contrast. At small flip angles, the fat lost this landmark role and imaged with a signal intensity comparable to that of the liver.

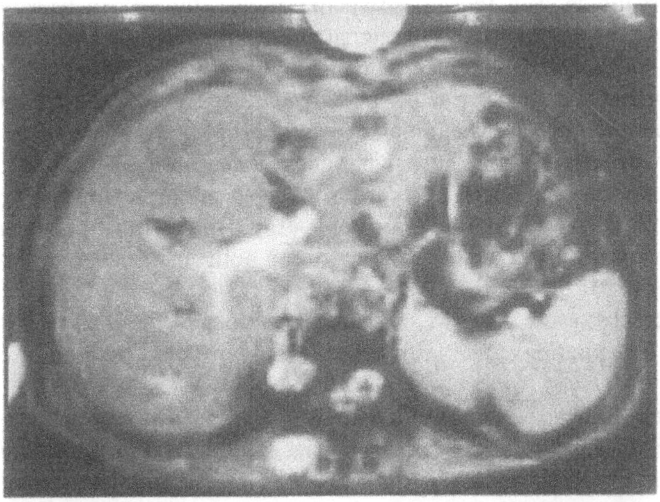

a

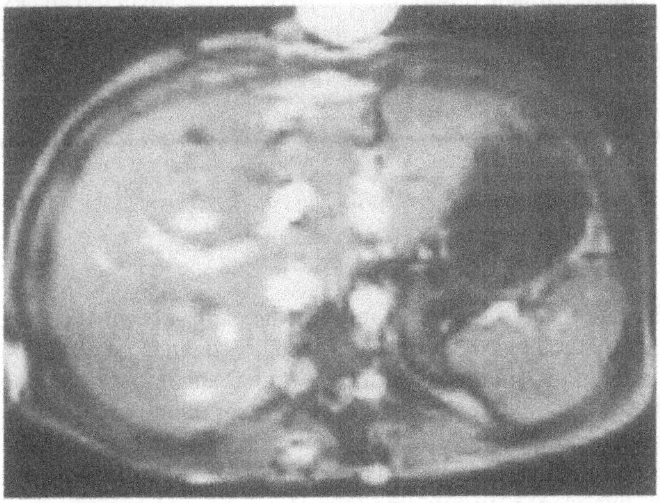

b

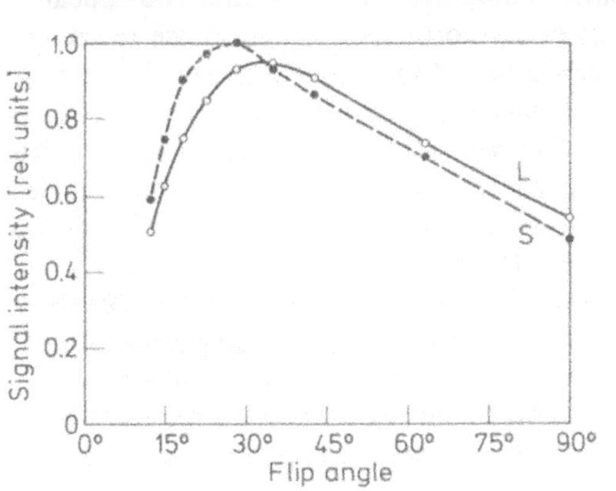

c

Fig. 4a–c. Axial MR scan using FLASH sequence (TR 80 ms, TE 16 ms) through upper abdomen of healthy volunteer. **a** Small flip angle. **b** Large flip angle. **c** Signal course with variation of flip angle; signal intensities here, as in following curves, are given in units relative to largest value. *L*, liver; *S*, spleen

Comparison of the organs showed that, at small flip angles, the spleen usually appeared brighter than the liver and surpassed the signal intensity of the fatty tissue. At large flip angles, the signal intensity of the liver, by contrast, was slightly higher.

The dependent relation between the characteristic signal courses of liver and spleen and the flip angles is presented in Fig. 4c. The initial increase for the spleen was typically steeper than for the liver, which explains the more signal-dense image at small flip angles, and the signal peaked at a smaller flip angle. Furthermore, the spleen peak was usually higher than that of the liver. In the intermediate flip angle range, the contrast between spleen and liver curves reversed, the signal difference between both curves at larger flip angles being relatively slight.

The steeper initial increase of the spleen curve suggests a longer T2; the smaller Ernst angle, a longer T1. This finding agrees with the values reported in the literature (*Moss* et al. 1983).

One important difference from acquisition with spin-echo sequences was the delineation of the large vessels. They appeared bright at small (Fig. 4a) and large (Fig. 4b) flip angles, with pronounced pulsation artifacts in the direction of the phase-encoding gradient. Both effects were more strongly pronounced at large than at small flip angles. The pulsation artifacts interfered particularly with the demonstration of the head of the pancreas, the left lobe of the liver, and the paravascular lymph nodes. Nevertheless, their direction could be varied by rotating the phase-encoding gradient (Fig. 6b, c).

5.2 Focal Liver Lesions: Comparison of Methods

5.2.1 Benign Masses

The hemangiomas, which were located predominantly in the right lobe of the liver, ranged from 4 to 8 cm in diameter. On US, five showed a clearly delineated, uniform, echo-dense structure; one hemangioma was uniformly more echo-poor than the surrounding liver (Fig. 5a); two had mixed echo texture with predominantly echo-dense areas and were clearly defined against the hepatic tissue. On plain CT, five of the hemangiomas were imaged as clearly delineated hypodense foci, one was hyperdense compared to the markedly hypodense surrounding liver (Fig. 5b), and two appeared as clearly delineated foci with punctiform or restiform central hypodense areas. On sequential CT, all hemangiomas showed localized punctiform areas of intensified density, predominantly at the periphery. The size of these areas gradually increased until they were confluent. On MRI, as on US and CT, they were clearly delineated, usually with a homogeneous structure. All hemangiomas appeared signal-intense at small flip angles (Fig. 5c, d). Four showed contrast reversal at intermediate flip angles and were darker than the surrounding liver at large flip angles (Table 3).

On US, an echinococcus cyst in the left lobe of the liver (Fig. 6a) imaged as echo-poor structures with surrounding echo-heterogeneous areas; no capsule could be identified. On CT, a mass with approximately water-isodense contents and a few septa was found. On MRI (Fig. 6b – d), this focus was clearly defined and again showed contrast reversal between small and large flip angles (Table 3). The inhomogeneity and the delineation of the lesion corresponded approximately to the CT scan. A capsule, however, could be identified, particularly at small flip angles.

Table 3. Analysis of signal courses of focal lesions with FLASH MRI

Focal change	Contrast with small flip angle	Contrast reversal	
		Yes	No
Liver			
Hemangioma	b	4 / 8	4 / 8
Echinococcus cysts	b	1 / 1	
FNH	b	1 / 1	
Gummata	b	1 / 1	
Metastasis	b	5 / 8	3 / 8
Primary hepatocellular carcinoma			
without hemochromatosis	± 0		2 / 2
with hemochromatosis	b		3 / 3
Lymphatic infiltration[a]	b	1 / 5	4 / 5
Spleen			
Lymphatic infiltration[a]	d		11 / 11
Fresh infarct	b		3 / 3
Old infarct	d		1 / 1
Leukosis	d		1 / 1
Sarcoidosis	d		1 / 1

b, focal lesion brighter than surrounding tissue; d, focal lesion darker than surrounding tissue
[a] One lesion not detected by FLASH MR imaging

In one female patient with focal nodular hyperplasia (FNH) of the liver, US showed a discrete echo-enhanced focus (diameter 12 cm) localized posteriorly in the right lobe of the liver. On plain CT (Fig. 7a) this focus appeared hypodense, on sequential CT as a massive, transitory enhancement of density in the arterial phase, which is characteristic for FNH. On MRI (Fig. 7b - c), this focus was also uniformly structured with a smooth margin. Furthermore, compared to the rest of the hepatic tissue it showed contrast reversal, with intense signal at small flip angles and weaker signal at large flip angles (Table 3).

In one patient with luetic gummata, multiple echo-poor, poorly defined foci were seen on US. These foci were hypodense against the hepatic tissue on CT, and showed no appreciable density enhancement on sequential CT. On MRI, they appeared as areas of slight signal enhancement and could barely be differentiated at small flip angles (Table 3).

5.2.2 Malignant Foci

US, CT, and MRI were equally effective for the demonstration of liver metastases. On US, the lesions were usually echo-poor (Fig. 8a) or cocardiform and ranged from 1.5 to 4 cm in diameter. On CT, they were all hypodense and hypovascularized, except for one metastasis from a carcinoid tumor. On MRI, all metastases were detected and imaged as signal-dense at small flip angles (Fig. 8b, left). Contrast reversal, with intense signal at small flip angles and weak signal at large flip angles, appeared in five of eight patients (Fig. 8b, c, Table 3).

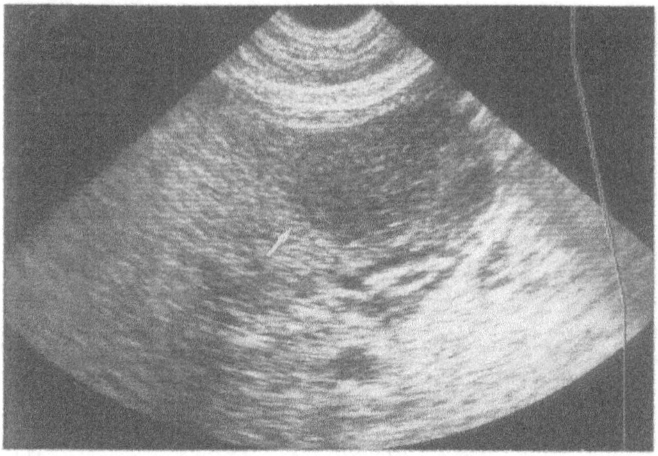

a

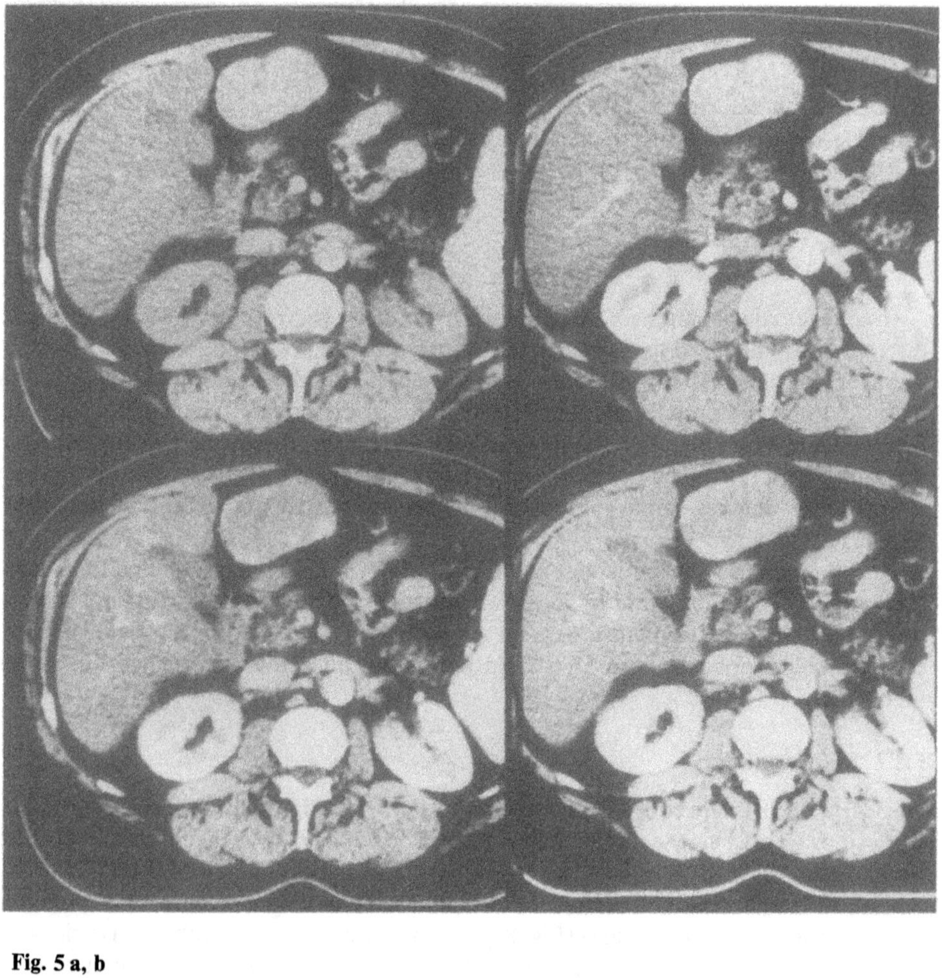

b

Fig. 5 a, b

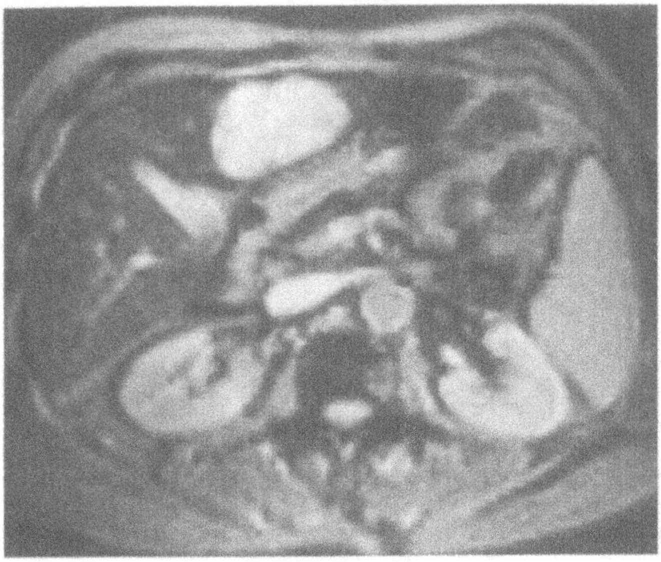

c

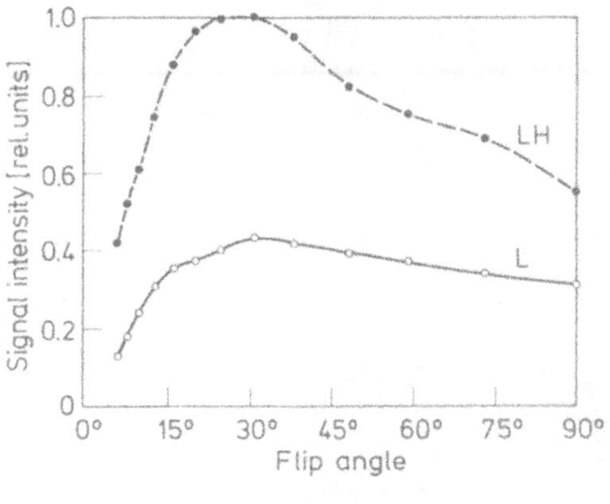

d

Fig. 5a–d. Hemangioma in left liver lobe. **a** Transverse US scan of upper abdomen; large echo-poor tumor (*arrow*) 6 cm in diameter in left lobe of liver. **b** Axial sequential CT scans. Plain CT (*upper left*): hyperdense focus in left lobe of hypodense liver. After bolus injection of contrast medium, punctiform, peripheral intensification of density (*upper right*: 10 s after injection), which gradually increased in size (*lower left*: 20 s after injection; *lower right*: 80 s after injection). **c** Axial MR scan (small flip angle): clearly delineated, signal-dense mass in left lobe of liver. **d** Signal course of hemangioma (*LH*) and surrounding hepatic tissue (*L*): signal intensity of hemangioma higher than that of liver at all flip angles; no contrast reversal in intermediate range of flip angles

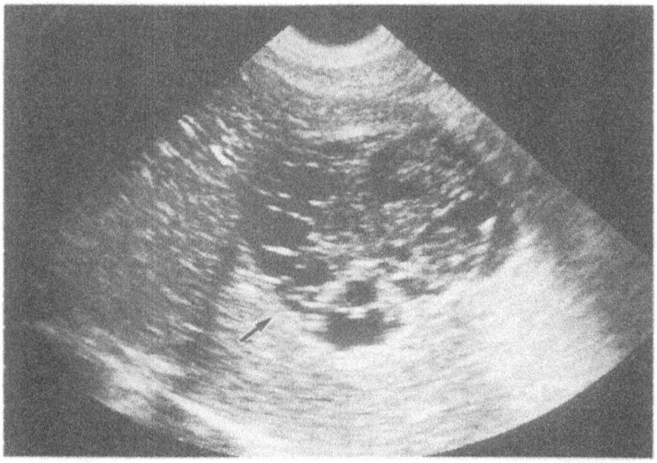

a

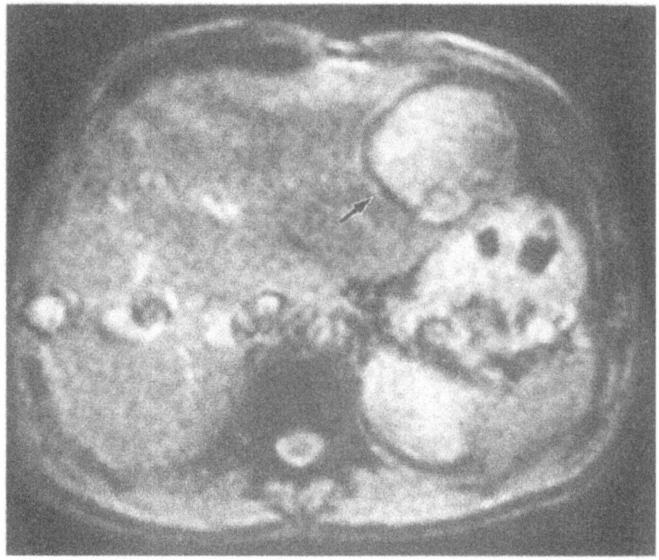

b

Fig. 6a–d. Echinococcus cyst (*arrow*) in left lobe of liver. **a** Transverse US scan of upper abdomen: heterogeneous, echo-poor mass in left lobe of liver with dorsal echo enhancement. **b** Axial MR scan (small flip angle): signal-dense cyst in left lobe of liver with round foci; signal-poor capsule. By rotating phase-encoding gradient, pulsation artifacts run horizontally and therefore do not interfere with imaging of left lobe of liver. **c** Axial MR scan (large flip angle): signal-poor cyst, relatively signal-dense capsule. **d** Signal course of echinococcus cyst (*LC*) and surrounding hepatic tissue (*L*): higher signal intensity of cyst at small flip angle, contrast reversal and lower signal intensity at large flip angle. Stronger contrast between cyst and hepatic tissue at large than at small flip angles

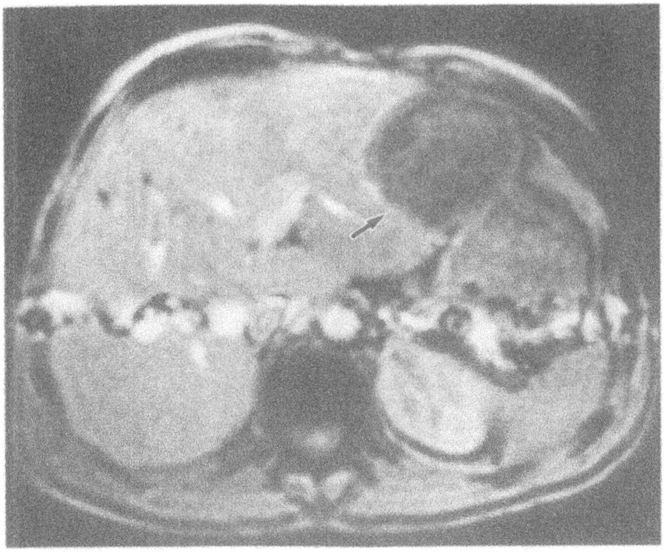

c

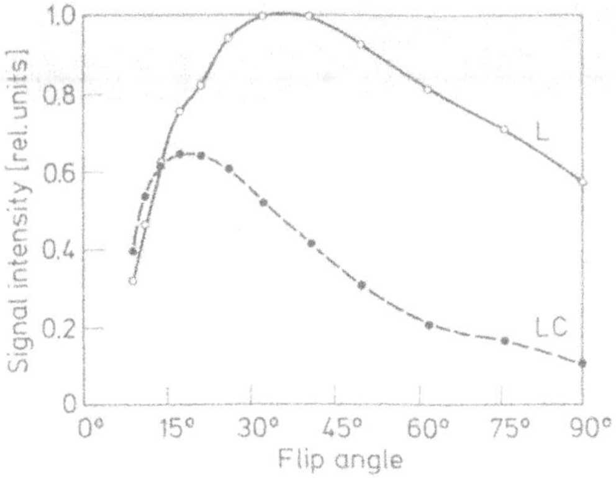

d

Fig. 6c, d

Solitary foci ranging from 4 to 8 cm in diameter were identified in the five patients with hepatocellular carcinoma. On US, two of these changes could not be clearly differentiated from the cirrhotic liver. The other three were more heterogeneous (Fig. 9a) than the rest of the hepatic tissue and could be discerned by virtue of their echo-poor rim and vascular displacement. All five tumors were hypodense against the hepatic tissue on plain CT, and showed heavy arterial vascularization on sequential CT (Fig. 10a). On MRI, two of the tumors had a signal intensity similar to that of the hepatic tissue at both small and large flip angles (Fig. 9b) and could be differentiated only by vascular displacement, inhomogeneity, or adjacent reaction. Three tumors contrasted well with the surrounding cirrhotic liver at all flip angles (Fig. 10b, Table 3); due to iron deposition, the liver parenchyma showed markedly diminished signal intensity.

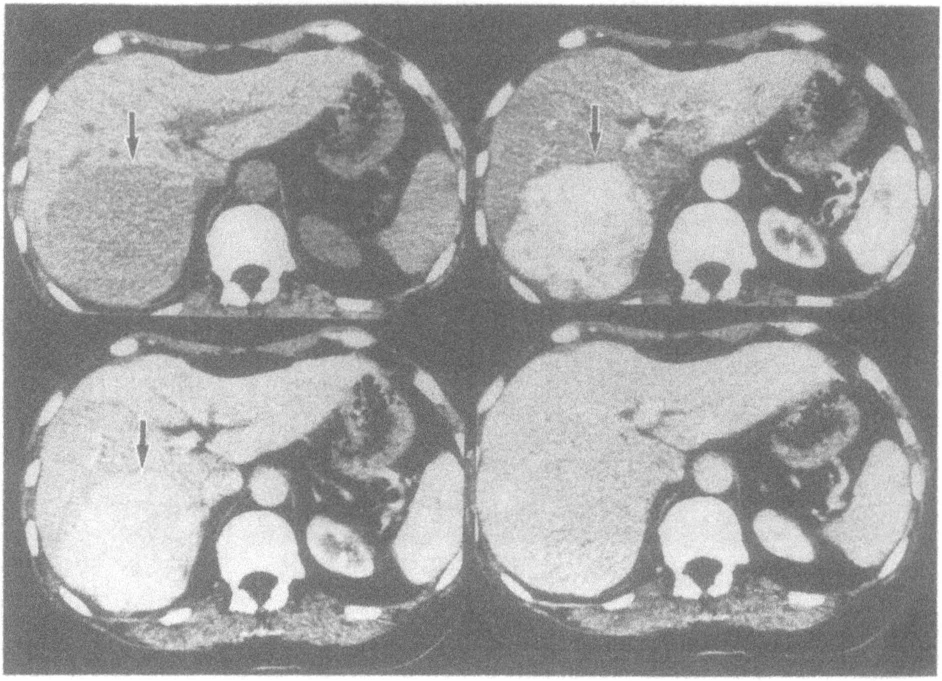

a

Fig. 7a–c. Focal nodular hyperplasia (*arrow*) in right lobe of liver. **a** Axial sequential CT scans. *Upper left*: plain CT; *upper right*: contrast-enhanced CT 10 s after injection, *lower left*: 20 s after injection; *lower right*: 60 s after injection. Plain CT shows mildly hypodense focus. Massive density enhancement in arterial phase with subsequent fast decline. **b** Axial MR scan (small flip angle): signal-dense, homogeneous mass, no capsule. **c** Axial MR scan (large flip angle): signal-poor mass

On US, six patients with lymphomatous involvement of the liver showed echo-poor foci ranging from 1.5 to 9 cm in diameter. In one patient with low-grade malignant lymphoma, the unaltered vascular architecture of the liver and the unimpaired course of both branches of the portal and the hepatic veins through the lesion were striking. On plain CT, this focus was hypodense, on sequential CT (Fig. 11a) it showed pronounced arterial density enhancement and was clearly defined in the venous phase. Three other liver lesions in Hodgkin's disease were also hypodense against the hepatic tissue and, after administration of contrast medium, showed circular density enhancement. The other two echo-poor masses demonstrated by US could not be identified on CT. Five of the six lymphomas could be confirmed by MRI. They appeared signal-intense at small flip angles (Fig. 11b, c); in only one case was there contrast reversal at large flip angles (Table 3).

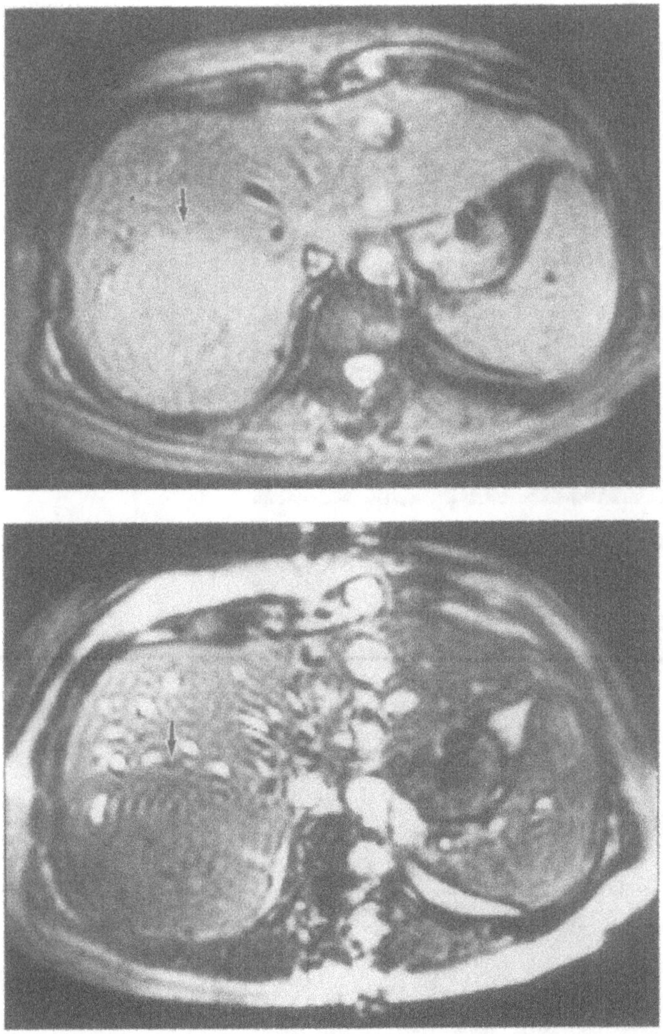

b

c

Fig. 7b, c

5.3 Focal Spleen Lesions: Comparison of Methods

5.3.1 Lymphatic Infiltration

Focal lymphatic infiltration of the spleen was demonstrated by at least one imaging method in 12 of 18 patients with confirmed malignant lymphoma (Table 4). The infiltrate was found predominantly in normal or slightly enlarged organs with a longitudinal diameter of 14 cm or less.

In 10 patients, the lesions were first detected on US. In eight of these cases they were more echo-poor than the surrounding organ (Figs. 12a, 13a), in two cases (both non-Hodgkin's lymphoma), homogeneous with an echo-poor rim. In seven of these

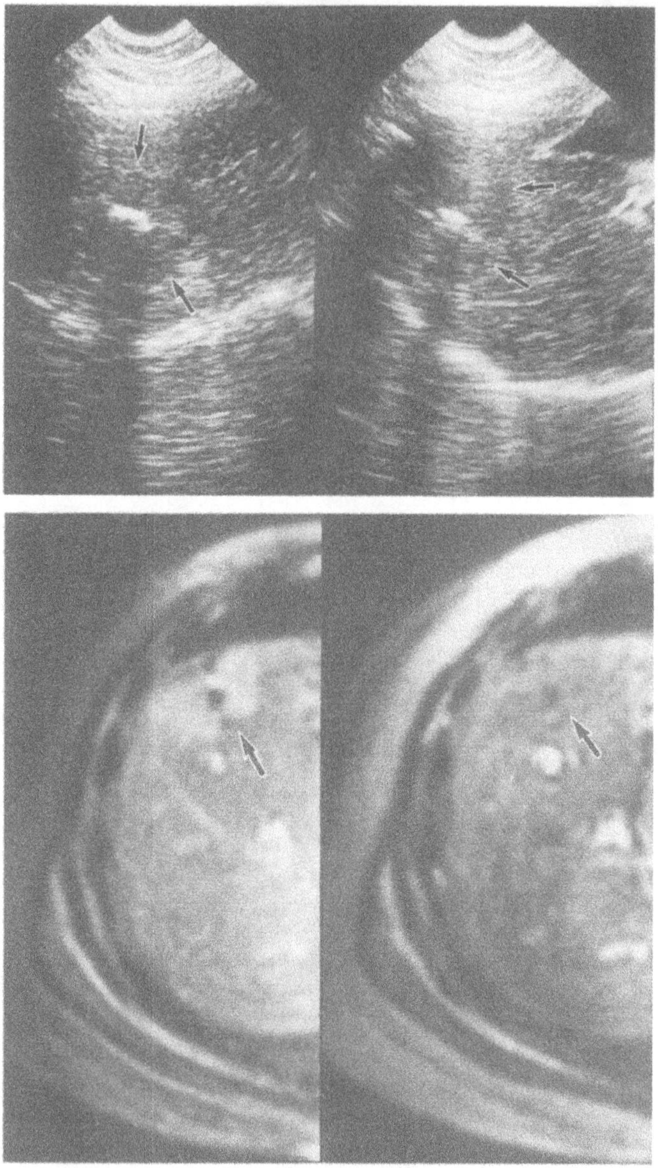

a

b

Fig. 8a–c. Metastasis from breast cancer (*arrows*) in right lobe of liver. **a** Subcostal US scan: echo-poor liver focus with echo-dense center and dorsal echo attenuation. **b** Axial MR scan (*left*: small flip angle, *right*: large flip angle): metastasis signal-intense at small flip angle and mildly signal-poor at large flip angle. Central, signal-poor structure at both flip angles corresponds with central calcification. **c** Signal course of metastasis (*LM*) and surrounding hepatic tissue (*L*): Contrast reversal at intermediate flip angles

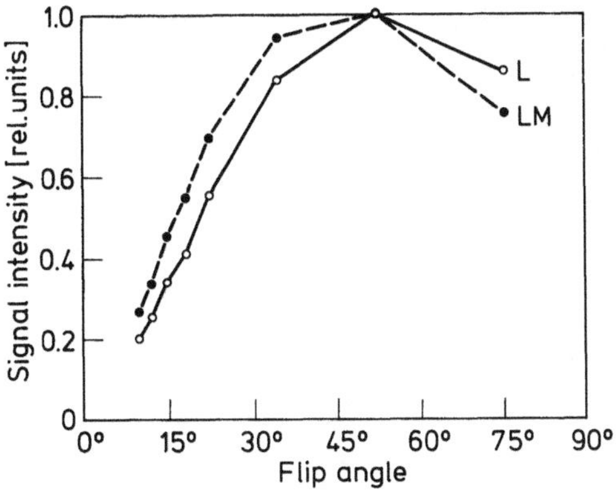

c

Fig. 8c

Table 4. Focal changes of spleen on US, CT, and MRI (number of patients in parentheses)

Spleen finding	US	CT	MRI
Lymphatic infiltrate (12)	Echo-poor focus or echo-homogeneous focus with echo-poor rim (10)	Hypodense focus in plain CT and / or diminished enhancement in sequential CT (9)	Focus with lower intensity (9)
		Normal (1)	Normal (1)
	Normal (2)	Normal (2)	Focus with lower intensity (2)
Leukemic infiltrate (1)	Echo-dense, later echo-poor focus	Normal, later hypodense focus	Focus with lower intensity
Involvement from sarcoidosis (1)	Echo-poor focus	Hypodense focus with diminished enhancement	Focus with lower intensity
Fresh splenic infarction (3)	Echo-poor focus (3)	Hypodense focus with minimal enhancement (3)	Focus with higher intensity (3)
Old infarct (1)	Echo-dense focus	Normal	Focus with lower intensity

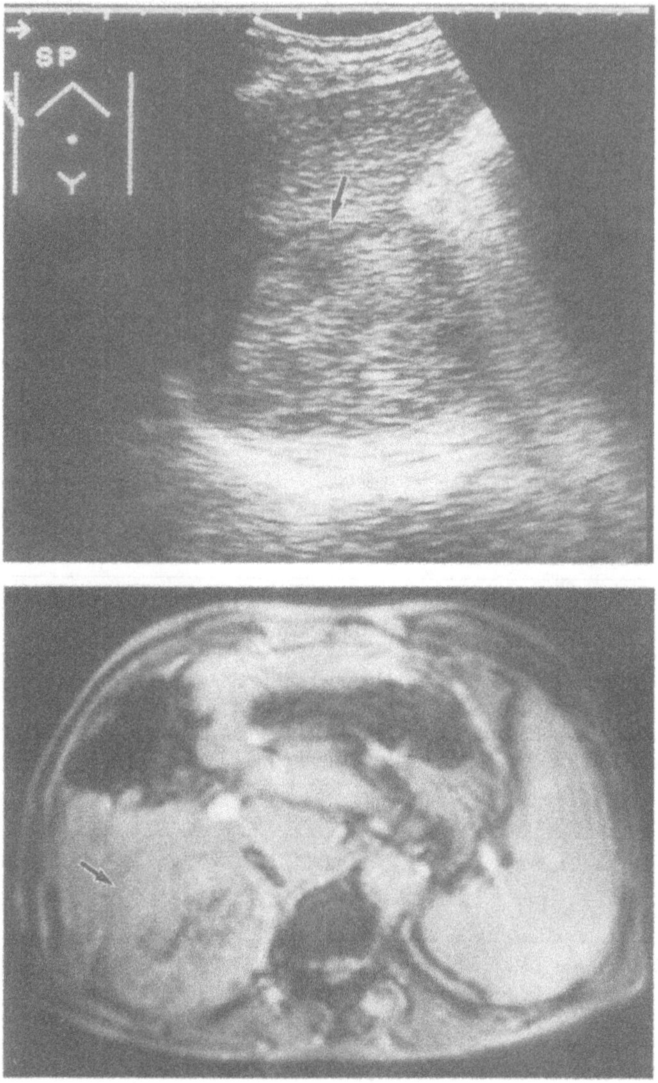

a

b

Fig. 9a, b. Hepatocellular carcinoma (*arrow*) in right lobe of liver. **a** Intercostal US scan: echo-heterogeneous tumor at underside of right lobe of liver. **b** Axial MR scan (intermediate flip angle): irregularly structured tumor dorsally in right lobe of liver, signal intensity similar to surrounding hepatic tissue; thin, barely discernible, signal-poor capsule; compression of inferior vena cava

10 patients, a corresponding hypodense area was found on plain CT and diminished enhancement on sequential CT (Fig. 12b). In three, the spleen was homogeneous on plain CT (Fig. 13b). In two of these three patients, a focus with diminished enhancement was demonstrated by sequential CT (Fig. 13b). Nine of ten lesions were therefore identified by sequential CT.

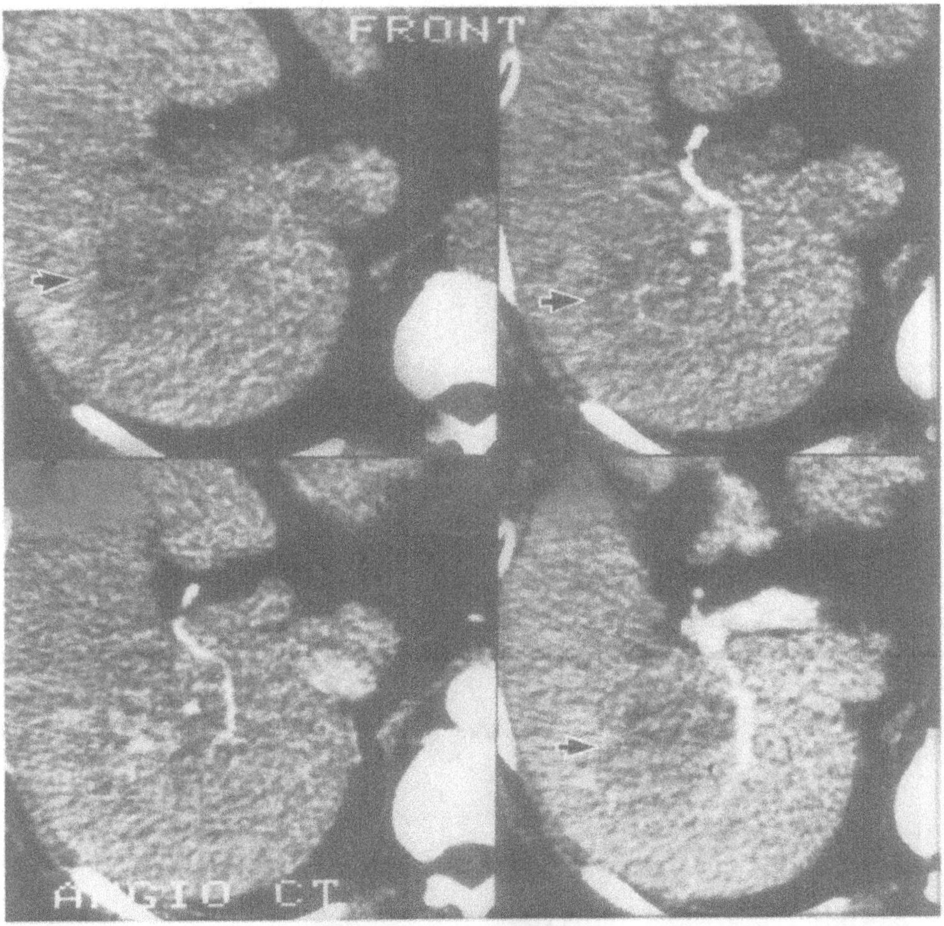

a

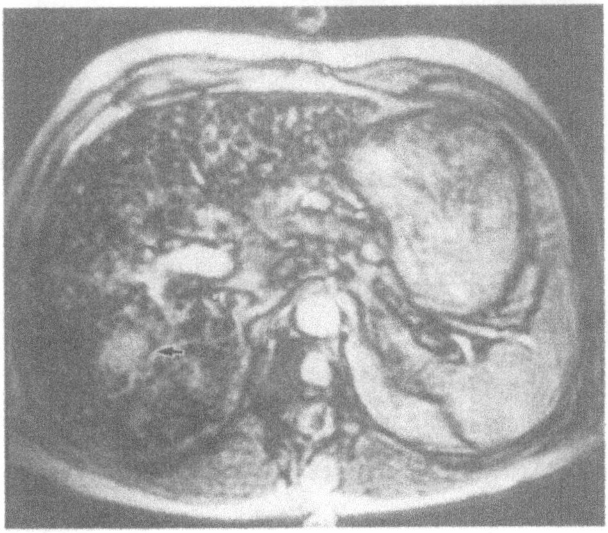

b

Fig. 10a, b. Hepatocellular carcinoma (*arrow*) in right lobe of liver in patient with liver cirrhosis and hemochromatosis. **a** Axial sequential CT scans. On plain CT (*upper left*), hypodense mass in right lobe of liver; pronounced enhancement in arterial phase 10 s (*upper right*) and 15 s (*lower left*) after injection of contrast medium; hypodense focus in portovenous phase (*lower right*). **b** Axial MR scan (intermediate flip angle): liver signal strikingly weak due to hemochromatosis, signal-dense tumor in right lobe of liver

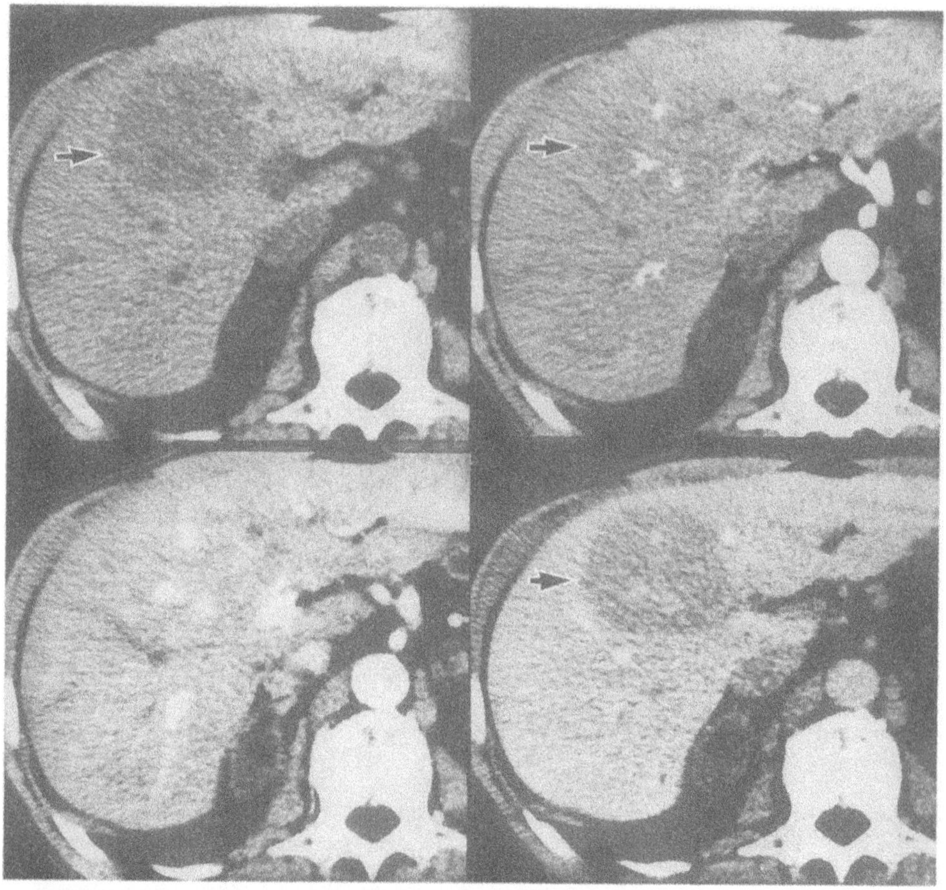

a

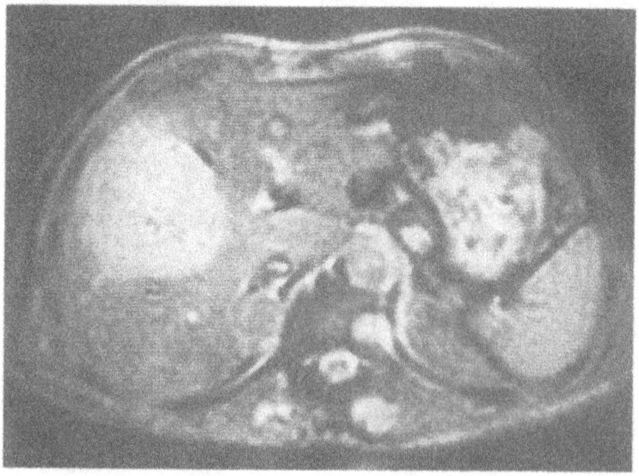

b

Fig. 11a–c. Low-grade malignant lymphoma of liver (*arrow*). **a** Axial sequential CT scans. On plain CT (*upper left*), hypodense focus in right lobe of liver; 5 s after injection of contrast medium (*upper right*), arterial density enhancement; pronounced hypodense imaging of focus in portovenous phase (*lower right*). Vascular structure of liver not appreciably impaired by tumor. **b** Axial MR scan (small flip angle): homogeneous signal-dense mass in right lobe of liver. **c** Signal course of lymphatic infiltrate (*LI*) and surrounding hepatic tissue (*L*): higher signal intensity of lymphatic infiltrate at all flip angles; no contrast reversal

c

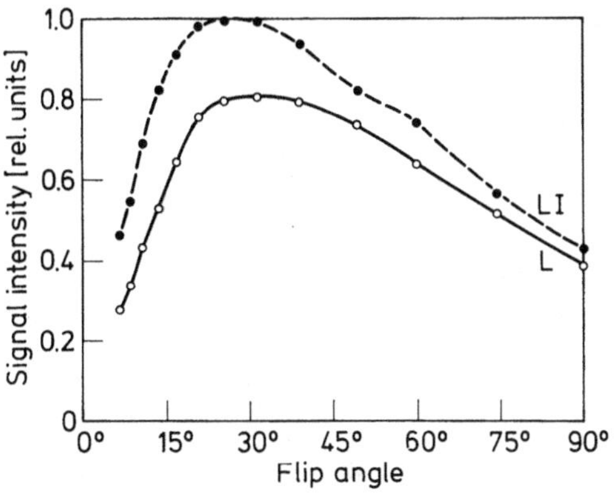

Fig. 11c

Table 5. Demonstrability of focal lymphatic involvement of spleen by US, CT, and MRI ($n = 12$)

Demonstrability	US	CT		MRI
		Plain	Sequential	
None	2	5	3	1
Poor	1	2	0	0
Moderate	6	2	5	3
Good	3	3	4	8

Corresponding signal-poor areas (Figs. 12c, 13d), compared to the surrounding spleen, were found on MRI. These areas were demonstrated at all flip angles (Fig. 12d, Table 3) but were best imaged at small to intermediate flip angles. In the cases with subsequent splenectomy, the configuration as seen on MRI was similar to that of the actual lesion (Figs. 12e, 13c).

As Table 5 shows, MRI was superior to US and sequential CT for the demonstration of circumscribed infiltrations of the spleen. Plain CT gave the worst results.

Whereas in one case a small circumscribed infiltration of a non-Hodgkin's lymphoma could be detected only by US (Table 4), in two patients circumscribed lymphatic involvement was detected only by MRI (Table 4). In one of these cases, lymphatic involvement of the liver was demonstrated by all methods; a circumscribed change of the spleen initially only by MRI. Three months later, the characteristic foci confirming the diagnosis of lymphatic involvement of the spleen were also seen on US and CT. In the second case with negative US and sequential CT findings, MRI showed a signal-poor focus; subsequent splenectomy revealed diffuse lymphatic involvement.

In one patient, lymphatic infiltration was initially visualized by all three methods. After chemotherapy, the circumscribed change disappeared on US and sequential CT. The persistence of the focus on MRI, however, indicated residual tumorous tissue; an echo-poor focus of the liver appearing for the first time on US also argued against remission of the disease.

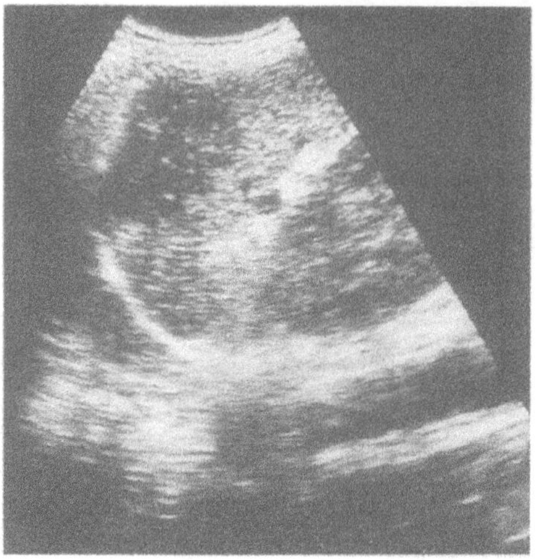

a

Fig. 12a–e. Splenic infiltrate (*arrow*) in Hodgkin's disease. **a** Longitudinal US scan: echo-poor focus in subdiaphragmatic parts of spleen. **b** Axial sequential CT scan: focus (hypodense area) poorly demonstrated on plain CT (*upper left*), but clearly differentiated on sequential CT. *Upper right:* 66 s after injection; *lower left:* 80 s after injection; *lower right:* 94 s after injection. **c** Axial MR scan (small to intermediate flip angle): signal-poor area. **d** Signal course of splenic infiltrate (*SI*) and surrounding spleen (*S*): low signal intensity of focus at all flip angles, focus best imaged at small to intermediate angles. **e** Gross specimen: distribution pattern of infiltrates on CT and MRI corresponds well to findings in resected spleen

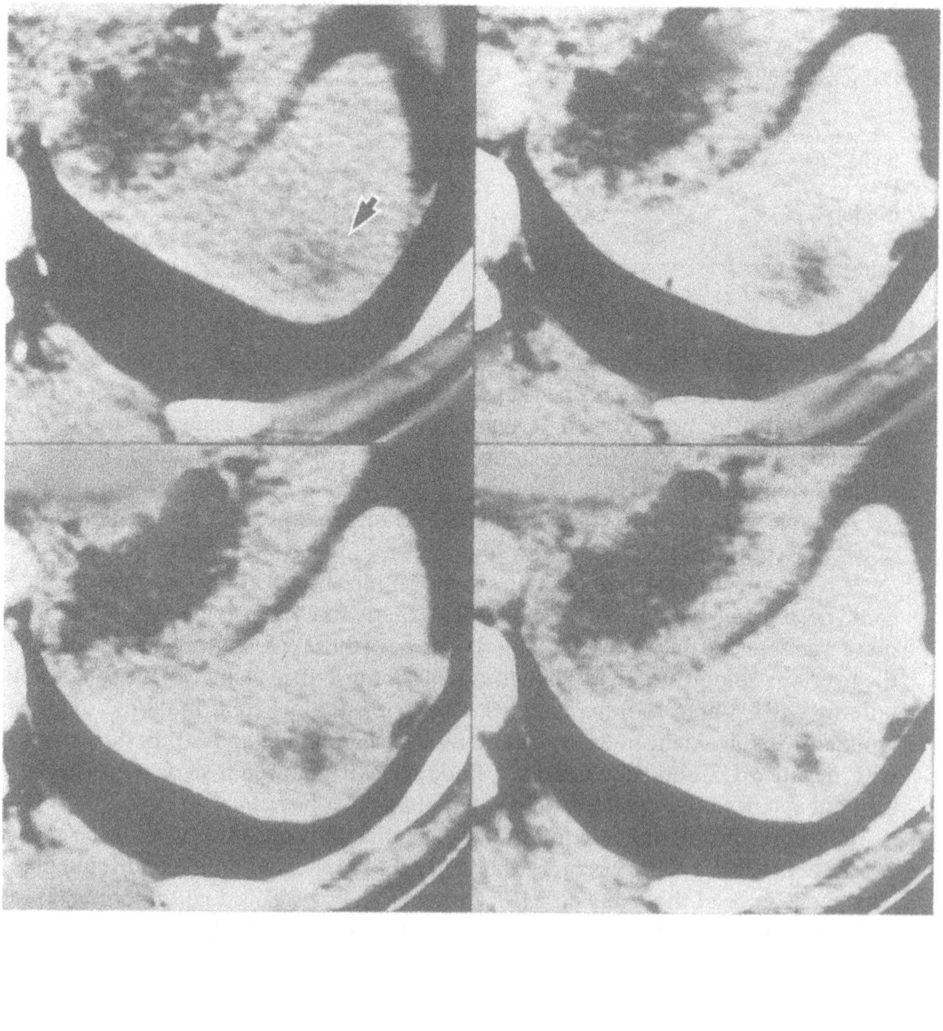

b

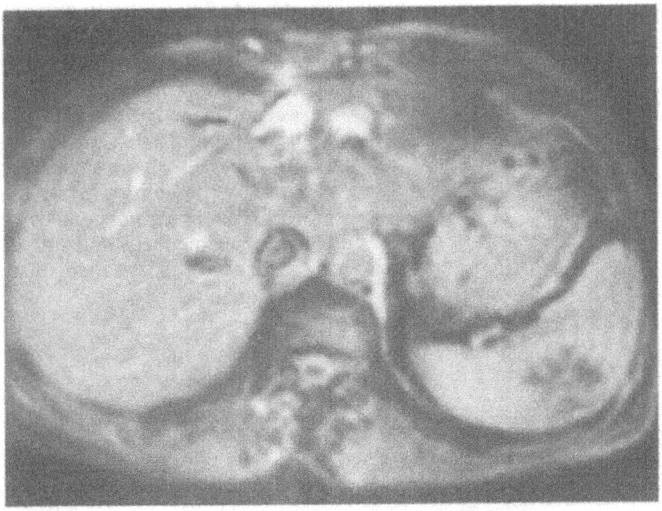

c

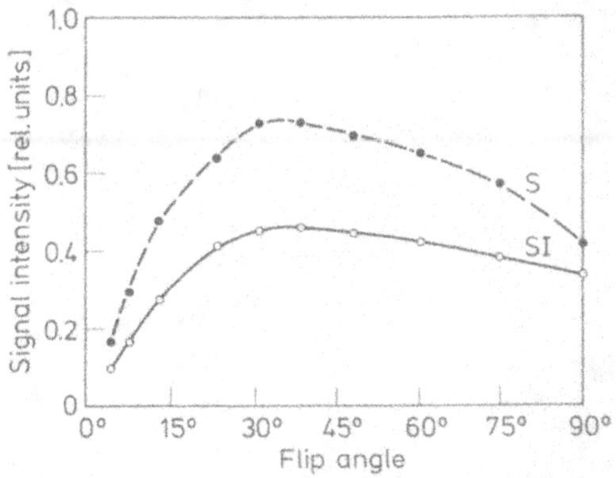
Signal intensity [rel. units]
1.0
0.8
0.6
0.4
0.2
0
S
SI
0° 15° 30° 45° 60° 75° 90°
Flip angle

d

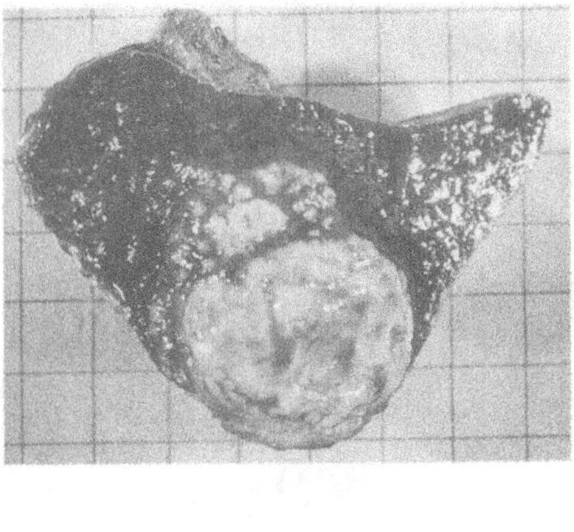

e

Fig. 12c–e

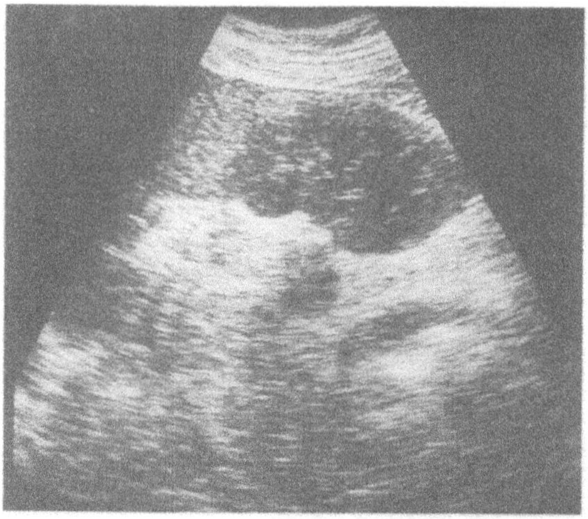

a

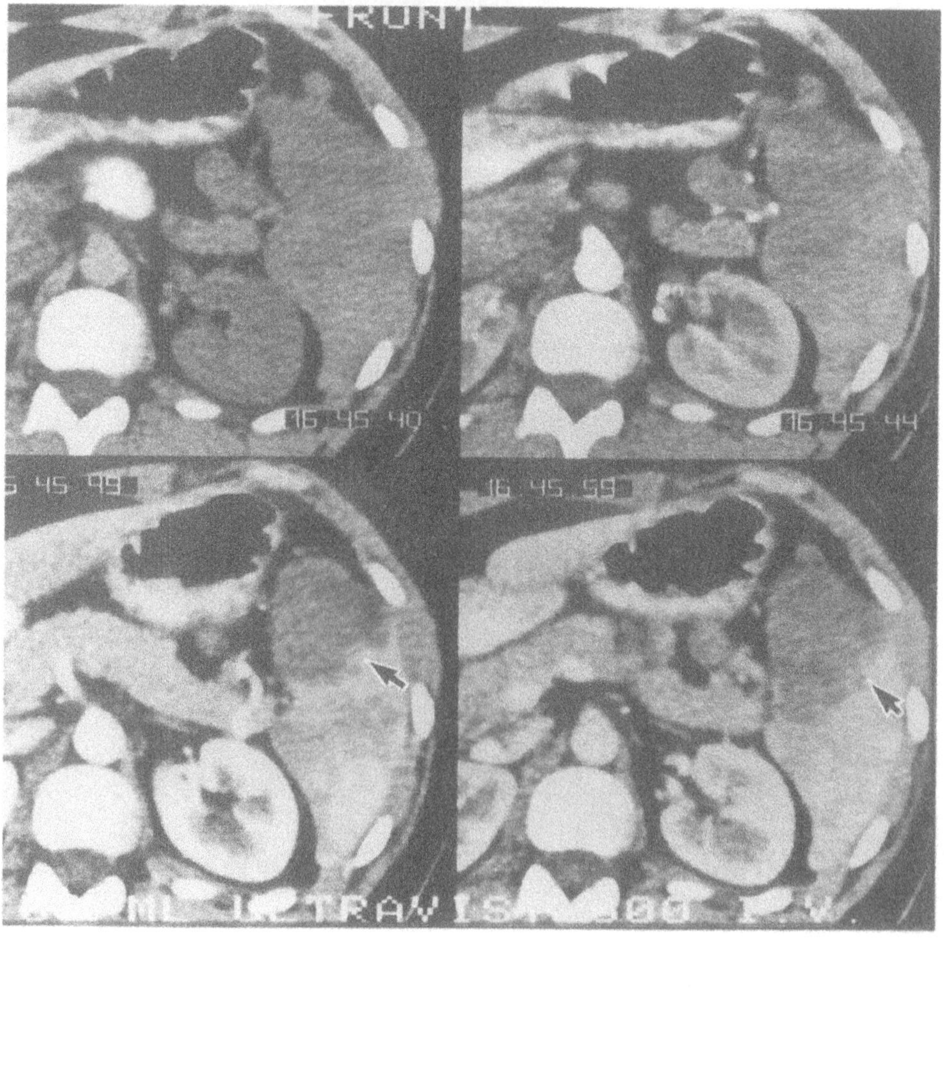

b

Fig. 13a–d. Splenic infiltrate (*arrow*) in Hodgkin's disease. **a** US scan: echopoor area at inferior pole of enlarged organ. **b** Axial sequential CT scans. Lesion not imaged on plain CT (*upper left*); good contrast 9 s (*lower left*) and 19 s (*lower right*) after bolus injection of contrast medium. **c** Gross specimen. **d** Axial MR scan: good contrast between splenic focus and surrounding spleen on MRI with small to intermediate flip angle

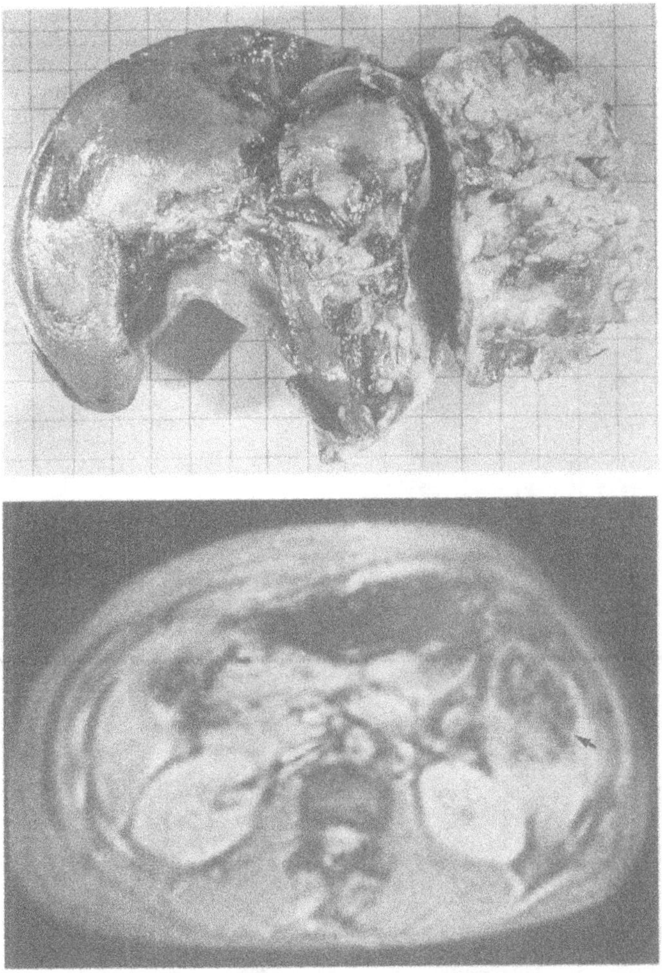

c

d

Fig. 13c, d

In six of 18 patients with malignant lymphoma, a focal change could not be detected by any imaging method. Whereas splenectomy revealed normal findings in one of these six cases, diffuse lymphatic involvement of the spleen was present on one other histologically confirmed case. In this case and in three of four patients with severe splenomegaly, the spleen appeared only slightly brighter, or even somewhat darker, than the liver on MRI at small flip angles, whereas it characteristically showed a higher signal intensity at these angles in healthy volunteers (see Sect. 5.1).

5.3.2 Focal Lesions of Nonlymphatic Etiology

In three cases, splenic foci signal-poor on MRI were not caused by lymphatic infiltrations (Tables 3, 4). In one patient (Fig. 14b), the focus represented splenic involvement by sarcoidosis, the configuration of which also resembled lymphatic involvement on US

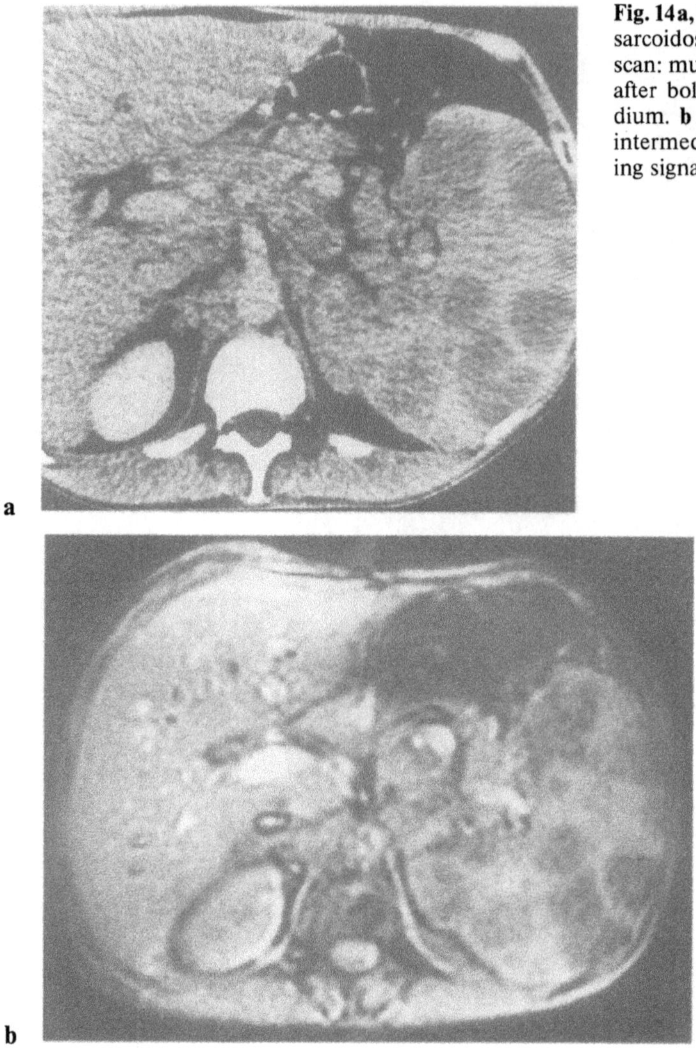

Fig. 14a, b. Involvement of spleen by sarcoidosis. **a** Axial sequential CT scan: multiple hypodense lesions 30 s after bolus injection of contrast medium. **b** Axial MR section (small to intermediate flip angle): corresponding signal-poor areas

(echo-poor foci) and CT (hypodense areas with diminished enhancement, Fig. 14a). In the second case, leukemic infiltration was present which was characterized on US initially by an echo-dense focus and later by an echo-poor focus. In the third patient, the lesion had a triangular configuration and was located in the periphery; in this case, the hyperintensity of the echo on US and the primary disease (recurrent atrial fibrillation) were indicative of an old splenic infarction.

Three patients with acute pain in the upper left abdomen (two with myeloproliferative syndrome, one with liver cirrhosis) were referred with the tentative diagnosis of fresh splenic infarction (Tables 3, 4). US showed echo-poor areas (Fig. 15a); CT, hypodense areas with mild contrast enhancement. MRI showed signal-dense areas at all flip angles, especially small and intermediate flip angles (Fig. 15b, c).

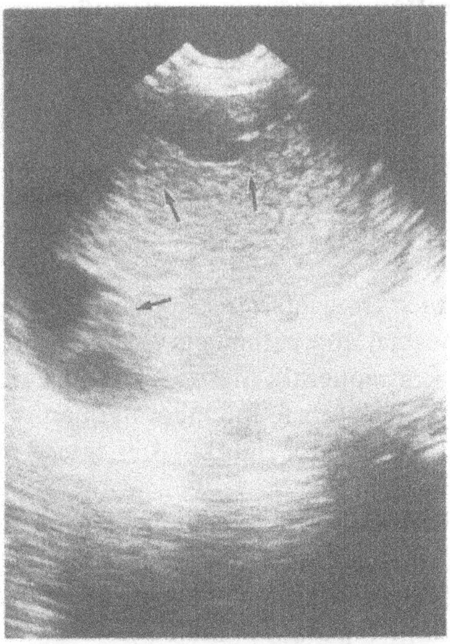

a

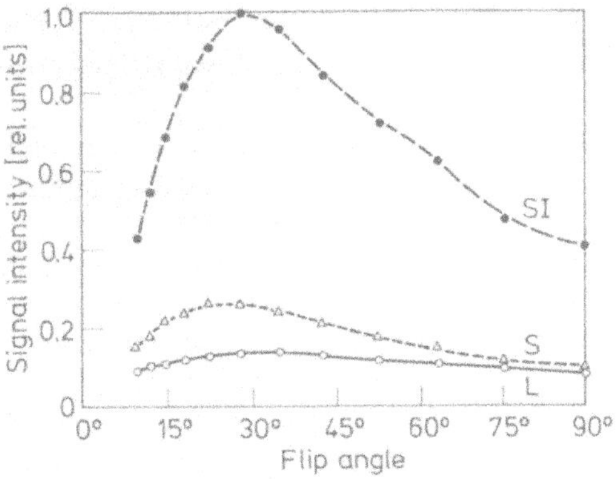

c

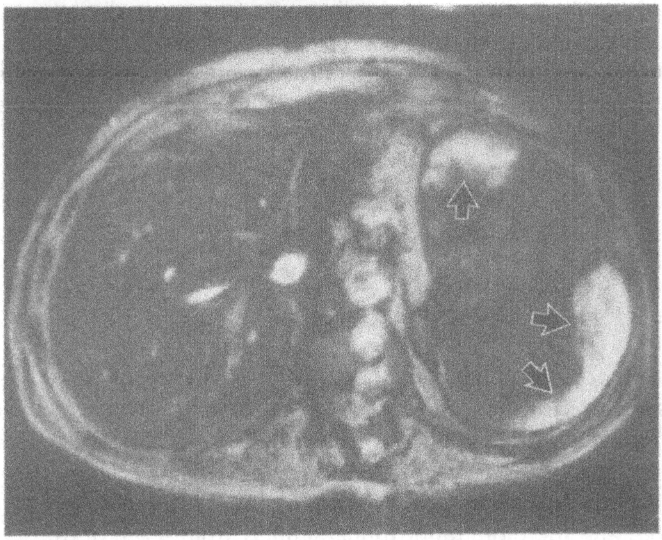

b

Fig. 15a–c. Recent splenic infarction (*arrows*) in patient with myeloproliferative syndrome. **a** Longitudinal US scan: extensive, echo-poor areas in periphery. **b** Axial MR section: signal-dense areas at small to intermediate flip angle. Striking weakness of signal in residual spleen and liver due to iron overload. **c** Signal course of infarct (*SI*), splenic tissue (*S*), and liver (*L*): signal intensity of foci higher than splenic tissue at all flip angles

5.4 Analysis of Signal Courses in Demonstration of Focal Hepatic and Splenic Lesions Using FLASH Sequences

Primary hepatocellular carcinoma in patients without hemochromatosis (Fig. 9b) imaged as inhomogeneous structures similar in signal intensity to the surrounding tissue (Table 3). All other lesions of the liver (Figs. 5c, 6b, 7b, 8b left, 11b), including primary hepatocellular carcinoma with hemochromatosis (Fig. 10b), appeared brighter than the surrounding tissue at small flip angles (Table 3).

Except for primary hepatocellular carcinoma, each group of liver lesions investigated showed contrast reversal phenomena between normal and pathologic tissue at intermediate flip angles (e.g., Figs. 6b - d, 7b, c, 8b, c). Consequently, these lesions appeared poor in signal at large flip angles. Nevertheless, this effect was found more frequently in liver metastases (five of eight) and liver hemangiomas (four of eight) than in lymphatic infiltrations of the liver (one of five) (Table 3).

Unlike the liver, no contrast reversal was found in focal lesions of the spleen. With the exception of fresh splenic infarctions (Fig. 15b, c), which appeared markedly brighter at all angles, all splenic lesions (Figs. 12c - d, 13d, 14b) showed a signal intensity lower than that of the surrounding tissue at both small and large flip angles (Table 3).

The demonstration of the focal changes of the liver was best at small flip angles (ca. 15° - 30°). With the exception of the echinococcus cyst (Fig. 6b - d), the contrast between focal lesion and surrounding tissue was generally slight at large flip angles. The best contrast between splenic lesion and surrounding tissue was achieved at small to intermediate flip angles (ca. 25° - 40°).

6 Discussion

The use of FLASH sequences enabled good demonstration of upper abdominal structures within a few seconds in suspended respiration and without the image quality being decreased by interference from respiratory artifacts, an advantage that is especially important at high field strengths (*Wood* and *Henkelman* 1986).

The signal courses of these sequences with variation of the flip angle show a peak (*Ernst* and *Anderson* 1966) and therefore differ fundamentally from those of the spin-echo and inversion-recovery sequences. Furthermore, image contrast depends primarily on the selection of the flip angle (*Edelman* et al. 1986; *Griebel* et al. 1987). T1-weighted scans are obtained at larger flip angles and T2*-weighted scans at small flip angles. An intensification of the somewhat mild T1 weighting can be achieved by shortening the echo delay time TE (*Edelman* et al. 1986). This, however, was not possible with our scanner at the time of this study.

The normal anatomy was best visualized at large flip angles, since, as with spin-echo sequences, the fatty tissue had the highest contrast against the organs of the upper abdomen on T1-weighted scans and, thereby, served as landmark. In this flip angle range, however, pulsation artifacts were the strongest and interfered with imaging of the head of the pancreas, the left lobe of the liver, and the paravascular lymph nodes.

Although FLASH sequences, on the whole, produce lower soft-tissue contrast than conventional sequences (*Bydder* and *Young* 1985b), hepatic and splenic lesions were extremely well demonstrated. Unlike the demonstration of the normal anatomy, the best contrast between focal lesion and surrounding tissue was achieved at small to intermediate flip angles. The extent to which tumor detection can be optimized by intensification of T1 weighting via shortening of TE (see above) must be established in future investigations.

Circumscribed liver diseases are demonstrated with similar sensitivity on US, CT, and MRI (*Hamm* et al. 1986; *Heiken* et al. 1985; *Moss* et al. 1984; *Baumann* et al. 1985; *Majewski* et al. 1984; *Alderson* et al. 1983; *Fiegler* et al. 1984; *Ebara* et al. 1986). Further reliable differentiation of solid hepatic foci is not possible on US and plain CT. After bolus administration of contrast medium sequential CT permits differential diagnosis in larger hemangiomas and, to a limited degree, in adenoma, FNH, and hepatocellular carcinoma (*Mathieu* et al. 1986; *Rogers* et al. 1981; *Takashima* et al. 1982; *Bree* et al. 1983; *Majewski* et al. 1983; *Nakao* et al. 1983; *Freeny* and *Marks* 1986). Hemangiomas can be differentiated from other hepatic foci only to a certain extent using conventional MRI sequences (*Stark* et al. 1985a; *Hamm* et al. 1986; *Baumann* et al. 1985; *Glazer* et al. 1985; *Ohtomo* et al. 1985). A reliable differentiation, especially of hepatocellular carcinoma and liver metastasis, is not possible. *Ebara* et al. 1986, however, demonstrated a capsule characteristic of hepatocellular carcinoma more frequently with MRI than with sequential CT.

In our study, on US, two hepatocellular carcinomas could not be differentiated from cirrhotic liver and four lesions were not reliably diagnosed as hemangiomas. US proved superior to CT and MRI with FLASH sequences for the detection of lymphomatous foci. Since sequential CT provided a characteristic picture of all hemangiomas, adjunctive angiography was necessary in only one case. All hepatocellular carcinomas showed typical enhancement in the arterial phase. FNH could also be diagnosed. The limits of the differential diagnosis proved to be arterial hypervascularized metastases or lymphomatous foci.

With the exception of one lymphomatous involvement of the liver, all foci detected on US or CT could also be demonstrated on MRI with FLASH sequences. FLASH sequences, like conventional MRI sequences (*Hamm* et al. 1986; *Moss* et al. 1984; *Baumann* et al. 1985), did not improve the differential diagnosis of focal liver lesions. Except for primary hepatocellular carcinoma in patients without hemochromatosis, all foci were signal-intense at small flip angles. The diagnostic significance of contrast reversal must also be assessed with caution. Except for primary hepatocellular carcinoma, this reversal was seen in all groups of lesions investigated.

There was a striking difference in the MRI appearance of primary hepatocellular carcinoma between patients with and those without increased iron deposition in the liver parenchyma. Whereas the carcinoma had a signal intensity similar to that of the surrounding hepatic tissue without increased iron deposition, it appeared bright with increased iron deposition. This is probably due to a marked reduction of the liver signal owing to shortening of T1 and T2 by the increased iron content, an effect which can also be observed on conventional sequences (*Stark* et al. 1985b; *Brown* et al. 1985).

Whereas many differential diagnoses must be considered in circumscribed changes of the liver, lymphatic involvement is by far the most frequent cause of circumscribed changes in the spleen (*Petersdorf* et al. 1983). Since such changes are rarely solitary and, consequently, imaging of the spleen is usually necessary in the context of the diagnosis of spread in cases with confirmed primary disease, sensitive demonstration of splenic involvement is more important than the differential diagnosis for the spleen. At present, however, sensitive demonstration is not ensured by US and sequential CT (*Bragg* et al. 1986; *Castellino* 1986). In those cases in which circumscribed lymphatic infiltration of the spleen can be demonstrated at all by these methods, they provide an extensively uniform picture which is also seen in our study: On US, demonstrable circumscribed lymphomatous infiltrations were usually echo-poor compared with the surrounding spleen, occasionally homogeneous with an echo-poor rim (*Lorenz* et al. 1983; *Solbiati* et al. 1983). On CT, such lesions were hypodense and showed only mild density enhancement after bolus injection of contrast medium (*Kurtz* 1986; *Anjou* et al. 1983).

Lymphatic foci in the spleen were demonstrated considerably better by MRI than by US and sequential CT; plain CT gave the worst results. On MRI with FLASH sequences, focal lymphatic infiltrates of the spleen were always characterized by signal-poor areas at all flip angles and were best detected at small to intermediate flip angles. The better visual contrast between lymphatic infiltration and surrounding splenic tissue on MRI, compared to US and sequential CT, may also explain why two of our cases of circumscribed involvement of the spleen were detected only by MRI.

Our studies, however, show that lymphatic involvement of the spleen can be present without demonstration of focal changes. In MRI, this phenomenon, known from US and CT, is partly due to unsatisfactory spatial resolution; splenic involvement by malignant lymphoma is frequently accompanied by the formation of multiple small foci of less than 1 cm in diameter (*Castellino* 1986; *Strijk* et al. 1985).

Furthermore, our preliminary findings tend to indicate that, on FLASH MRI at small flip angles, lymphatic infiltration can result in a signal intensity of the whole spleen that is lower than or similar to that of the liver. The normal spleen was typically brighter than the liver at that setting. This hypothesis, however, must be confirmed in larger patient populations, as with analogous studies of US (*Sommer* et al. 1984) and CT (*Kurtz* 1986). Moreover, our findings show that the diagnosis of splenic involvement cannot be reliably established on the basis of spleen size. Like other authors (*Castellino* 1986; *Kadin* et al. 1971; *Kurtz* 1986), we have frequently found lymphatic infiltration in normal or slightly enlarged organs.

Focal splenic changes of nonlymphatic etiology are rarer than those caused by malignant lymphomas, but can be similar in appearance, especially on US and CT (*Anjou* et al. 1983; *Lorenz* et al. 1983; *Solbiati* et al. 1983). Whereas leukemic infiltration and splenic involvement from sarcoidosis could not be differentiated from lymphatic infiltration by any of the imaging methods, fresh splenic infarction, the most frequent nonlymphatic splenic lesion, produced a different picture, i. e., extremely signal-dense areas, on MRI. As is well known, the differential diagnosis cannot be reliably established by US and sequential CT (*Balcar* et al. 1984; *Lorenz* et al. 1983).

Old splenic infarctions also appeared as signal-poor foci on MRI, but as echo-dense foci on US. Since this US finding is extremely unusual for a lymphatic infiltrate (*Solbiati* et al. 1983), US and MRI together enable differentiation of the pathologic finding. Clear evaluation of cysts and areas of calcification in the spleen presents no problems on US and CT (*Anjou* et al. 1983; *Lorenz* et al. 1983; *Solbiati* et al. 1983). Since metastases of solid tumors and benign tumorous changes of the spleen are extremely rare (*Petersdorf* et al. 1983), we did not include them in our comparative studies.

On the whole, extensive differentiation of relevant focal changes of the spleen is possible by means of adjunctive MRI with FLASH sequences. The better demonstration of splenic foci and the greater sensitivity in the detection of lymphatic infiltration represent considerable progress in the imaging of the spleen.

Further studies will clarify whether the sensitivity of MRI in the detection of lymphatic infiltration of the spleen can be increased by use of surface coils and whether the MRI differential diagnosis of focal lesions of the liver can be improved by administration of contrast medium in FLASH sequences.

7 Summary

Fifteen healthy volunteers and 54 patients (liver study $n=30$, spleen study $n=24$) were examined with MRI using gradient-echo sequences (FLASH: TR 80 ms, TE 16 ms). Prior to MRI evaluation, all patients were examined by plain and sequential CT and by US; the diagnoses were confirmed by clinical examination or, when necessary, histologic assessment.

Good delineation of the upper abdominal structures could be achieved by FLASH sequences within a few seconds in suspended respiration and without the image quality being affected by interference from respiratory artifacts.

The contrast between these structures was essentially determined by the selection of the flip angle. The normal anatomy was best demonstrated using intermediate to large flip angles, since here the fatty tissue was more signal-dense than the organs of the upper abdomen and therefore served as landmark. In this flip angle range, however, pulsation artifacts perpendicular to the large vessels were strongest and interfered with the visualization of the head of the pancreas, the left lobe of the liver, and the paravascular lymph nodes. The best contrast between focal lesions and adjacent tissue was achieved at small to intermediate flip angles.

Comparison of US, sequential CT, and FLASH MRI revealed that they have similar sensitivity with respect to the demonstration of focal liver diseases. As with conventional MRI sequences, the differential diagnosis of focal lesions of the liver was not improved by FLASH sequences. At all flip angles, primary hepatocellular carcinoma in patients without increased iron deposition in the liver appeared as an inhomogeneous structure with a signal intensity similar to that of the liver. At small flip angles, all other liver lesions were more signal-dense than the adjacent tissue. With increasing flip angles, contrast reversal phenomena between lesion and liver parenchyma were observed in all diagnostic groups examined except the primary hepatocellular carcinomas, leading to signal-weak imaging of these lesions at large flip angles. The best delineation of liver lesions was found at small flip angles (ca. 15° - 30°).

For imaging of the spleen, MRI with FLASH sequences was clearly superior to US and sequential CT; the worst results were obtained with plain CT. Circumscribed lymphatic infiltrates, the most frequent focal change of the spleen, were imaged by FLASH with greater sensitivity and better contrast against the adjacent tissue. These infiltrates were always characterized by signal-poor areas at all flip angles and were best detected using small to intermediate flip angles (ca. 25° - 40°). By contrast, fresh splenic infarctions appeared on MRI as signal-dense changes and therefore, in contrast to the situation with US and CT, could be clearly differentiated from lymphatic involvement of the spleen.

References

Alderson PO, Adams DF, McNeil BJ, Sanders R, Siegelman SS et al. (1983) Computed tomography, ultrasound, and scintigraphy of the liver in patients with colon or breast carcinoma: a prospective comparison, Radiology 149: 225 - 230

Anjou A, Chollat L, Bret PM et al. (1983) Apport de la tomodensitometrie dans la pathologie splenique focalisee. Ann Radiol (Paris) 26 (4): 275 - 283

Balcar I, Seltzer SE, Davis BS et al. (1984) CT patterns of splenic infarction: a clinical and experimental study. Radiology 151: 723 - 729

Baumann R, Grodd W, Kurtz B (1985) Kernspintomographische Untersuchungen bei Erkrankungen der Leber. Fortschr. Röntgenstr. 142: 494 - 504

Bragg DG, Colby TV, Ward JH (1986) New concepts in the non-Hodgkin lymphomas: radiologic implications. Radiology 159: 289 - 304

Bree RL, Schwab RE, Neiman HL (1983) Solitary echogenic spot in the liver: is it diagnostic of a hemangioma? AJR 140: 41 - 45

Brown DW, Henkelman RM, Poon PY, Fisher MM (1985) Nuclear magnetic resonance study of iron overload in liver tissue. Magn Reson Imaging 3: 275 - 282

Bydder GM, Young IR (1985 a) MRI: clinical use of the inversion recovery sequence. J Comput Assist Tomogr 9 (4): 659 - 675

Bydder GM, Young IR (1985 b) Clinical use of the partial saturation and saturation revovery sequences in MR imaging. J Comput Assist Tomograph 9 (6): 1020 - 1032

Castellino RA (1986) Hodgkin disease: Practical concepts for the diagnostic radiologist. Radiology 159: 305 - 310

Ebara M, Ohto M, Watanabe Y et al. (1986) Diagnosis of small hepatocellular carcinoma: correlation of MR imaging and tumor histology studies. Radiology 159: 371 - 377

Edelman RR, Hahn PF, Buxton R, Wittenberg J et al. (1986) Rapid MR imaging with suspended respiration: clinical application in the liver. Radiology 161: 125 - 131

Ernst RR, Anderson WA (1966) Application of Fourier transform spectroscopy to magnetic resonance. Rev Sci Instrum 37: 93 - 102

Fiegler W, Schütz H, Claussen C, Schörner W, Felix R (1984) Herdförmige Lebererkrankungen. Fortschr. Röntgenstr. 141 (1): 71 - 74

Freeny PC, Marks WM (1986) Hepatic hemangioma: dynamic bolus CT. AJR 147: 711 - 719

Glazer GM, Aisen AM, Francis IR, Gyves JW et al. (1985) Hepatic cavernous hemangioma: magnetic resonance imaging. Radiology 155: 417 - 420

Griebel J, Hess CF, Kurtz B, Klose U, Küper K (1987) Erste Ergebnisse in der Diagnostik fokaler Leber- und Milzläsionen mittels Gradientenecho Sequenzen. Fortschr. Röntgenstr. 146 (1): 18 - 23

Haase A, Frahm J, Matthaei D, Hänicke W, Merboldt K-D (1986) FLASH imaging. Rapid NMR imaging using low flip-angle pulses. J Magn Reson 67: 258 - 266

Hamm B, Römer T, Friedrich M, Felix R, Wolf K-J (1986) Magnetische Resonanztomographie fokaler Leberläsionen im Vergleich zur Computertomographie und Sonographie. Fortschr. Röntgenstr. 144 (3): 278 - 286

Heiken JP, Lee JKT, Glazer HS, Ling D (1985) Hepatic metastases studied with MR and CT. Radiology 156: 423 - 427

Kadin ME, Glatstein E, Dorfman RF (1971) Clinicopathologic studies of 117 untreated patients subjected to laparatomy for the staging of Hodgkin's disease. Cancer 27: 1277 - 1285

Klose U, Deimling M, Griebel J, Schroth G (1986) Bestimmung der Kernspinrelaxationszeit T1 durch Gradientenecho Sequenzen. Medizinische Physik 1986, Lübeck, 87 - 94 17. Wissenschaftliche Tagung der Deutschen Gesellschaft für Medizinische Physik e.V.

Kurtz B (1986) Dynamische Computertomographie bei Lymphommanifestationen von Leber und Milz. Fortschr. Röntgenstr. 144 (2): 149 - 153

Lorenz R, Beyer D, Friedmann G, Moedder U (1983) Grenzen der Differenzierung fokaler Milzläsionen durch Sonographie und Computertomographie. Fortschr. Röntgenstr. 138 (4): 447 - 452

Majewski A, Hendrickx P, Brölsch C, Wiese H (1983) Computertomographische Densitometrie primärer Lebertumoren. Fortschr. Röntgenstr. 138 (1): 8 - 14

Majewski A, Gratz KF, Brölsch C, Gebel M (1984) Sonographic pattern of focal nodular hyperplasia of the liver. Eur J Radiol 4: 52 - 57

Mathieu D, Bruneton JN, Drouillard J, Pointreau CC, Vasile N (1986) Hepatic adenomas and focal nodular hyperplasia: dynamic CT study. Radiology 160: 53 - 58

Moss AA, Stark DD, Goldberg HI, Margulis AR (1983) Liver, gallbladder, alimentary tube, spleen, peritoneal cavity, and pancreas. In: Margulis AR et al. (eds) Clinical Magnetic Resonance Imaging. Radiology Research and Education Foundation, San Francisco, 185 - 207

Moss AA, Goldberg HI, Stark DB et al. (1984) Hepatic tumors: magnetic resonance and CT appearance. Radiology 150: 141 - 147

Nakao N, Miura K, Takayasu Y, Wada Y, Miura T (1983) CT angiography in hepatocellular carcinoma. J Comput Assist Tomogr 7 (5): 780 - 787

Ohtomo K, Itai Y, Furui S, Yashiro N et al. (1985) Hepatic tumors: differentiation by transverse relaxation time (T2) of magnetic resonance imaging. Radiology 155 : 421 - 423

Petersdorf RG, Adams RD, Braunwald E et al. (1983) Harrison's principles of internal medicine. McGraw Hill, New York, 301

Rogers JV, Mack LA, Freeny PC, Johnson ML, Sones PS (1981) Hepatic focal nodular hyperplasia: angiography, CT, sonography, and scintigraphy. AJR 137: 983 - 990

Runge VM, Clanton JA, Partain CL, James AE (1984) Respiratory gating in magnetic resonance imaging at 0.5 tesla. Radiology 151: 521 - 523

Solbiati L, Bossi MC, Bellotti E, Ravetto C, Montali G (1983) Focal lesions in the spleen: sonographic patterns and guided biopsy. AJR 140: 59 - 65

Sommer FG, Hoppe RT, Fellingham L et al. (1984) Spleen structure in Hodgkin disease: ultrasonic characterisation. Radiology 153: 219 - 222

Stark DD, Felder RC, Wittenberg J et al. (1985 a) MR imaging of cavernous hemangioma of the liver. AJR 145: 213 - 222

Stark DD, Moseley ME, Bacon BR et al. (1985 b) Magnetic resonance imaging and spectroscopy of hepatic iron overload. Radiology 154: 137 - 142

Stark DD, Wittenberg J, Edelman RR et al. (1986) Detection of hepatic metastases: analysis of pulse sequence performance in MR imaging. Radiology 159: 365 - 370

Strijk SP, Wagener DJT, Bogman MJJT et al. (1985) The spleen in Hodgkin disease: diagnostic value of CT. Radiology 154: 753 - 757

Takashima T, Matsui O, Suzuki M, Ida M (1982) Diagnosis and screening of small hepatocellular carcinomas. Radiology 145: 635 - 638

Van der Meulen P, Groen JP, Cuppen JJM (1985) Very fast imaging by field echos and small angle excitation. Magn Reson Imaging 3: 297 - 299

Wood ML, Henkelman RM (1986) The magnetic field dependence of the breathing artefact. Magn Reson Imaging 4: 387 - 392

Analysis of the Signal Intensity of FLASH and FISP Fast-Imaging Pulse Sequences*

S.H. Heywang[1], G. Koebrunner[2], and M.W. Bauer[1]

1 Introduction

Both long examination times and long acquisition times have been considered significant disadvantages in the routine clinical application of MRI. Since 1985 several so-called fast-imaging pulse sequences have been developed. A number of these pulse sequences, like fast low-angle shot imaging (FLASH) and fast imaging with steady precession (FISP), are based on a steady state, using very short repetition times (TR), very short echo times (TE) produced by gradient echos, and variable flip angles (*Oppelt* et al. 1986; *Weber* et al. 1986; *Frahm* et al. 1986; *Mills* et al. 1987; *Matthaei* et al. 1986; *Weber* and *Deimling* 1987; *Krestin* et al. 1986).

Compared to spin-echo (SE) or inversion-recovery (IR) sequences, it appears more difficult for the radiologist to achieve an understanding of the resulting contrast. This fundamental understanding is essential, however, for the correct choice of the imaging parameters (TR, TE, flip angle α), for the meaningful application of these pulse sequences and for the correct interpretation of the resulting images.

This paper presents an analysis of the contrast of FLASH and FISP sequences which should give better insight into the potential and the limitations of these pulse sequences.

---

* This study was supported by the Deutsche Krebshilfe e.V.

[1] Radiologische Klinik, Klinikum Großhadern (Dir.: Prof. Dr. Dr. h.c. J. Lissner), Universität München, Marchioninistraße 15, D-8000 München 70, FRG

[2] Siemens AG, Medizinische Technik, Richard-Strauss-Straße 76, D-8000 München 80, FRG

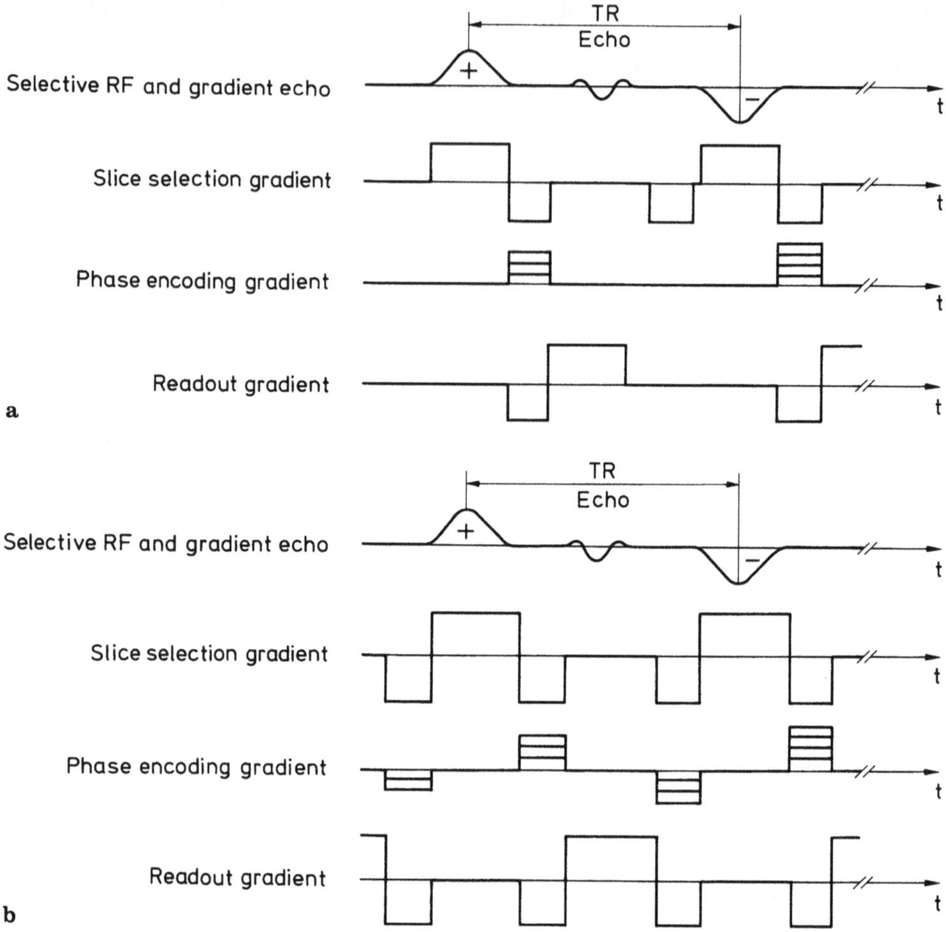

Fig. 1a, b. Pulse sequence schematics **(a)** for FLASH and **(b)** for FISP. (From *Oppelt* et al. 1986)

2 Theory

Both FLASH and FISP are so-called gradient-echo sequences, as illustrated in Fig. 1a,b.

They are determined by the repetition time TR, the echo time of the gradient echo TE and the flip angle of the radiofrequency (RF) excitation pulse (*Weber* et al. 1986 a, b; *Weber* and *Deimling* 1987).

The resulting signal intensity *I* can be approximated by the following equation, which is valid for phase-alternating RF excitation (*Weber* et al. 1986 b; *Mansfield* and *Morris* 1982):

$$I \sim \frac{\text{rho} \cdot [1 - \exp(\text{TR}/\text{T1})] \cdot \sin\alpha \cdot \exp(-\text{TE}/\text{T2}^*)}{[1 - \exp(-\text{TR}/\text{T1}) \cdot \cos\alpha] + \exp(-\text{TR}/\text{T2}) \cdot [\cos\alpha - \exp(-\text{TR}/\text{T1})]} \qquad (1)^3$$

where rho = proton density.

[3] Equations 1-3 are valid in an ideal system

Since for fast imaging TR is usually set short compared to T1, a steady state is obtained in the longitudinal direction. If TR is also significantly shorter than T2, steady state is possible in the transverse direction as well.

The potential steady state in the transverse direction is preserved for FISP by use of a special refocusing gradient, whereas it is destroyed for FLASH by a so-called spoiler gradient. Therefore a steady state in both the transverse and the longitudinal direction is possible for FISP, depending on the T1 and T2 of the tissue, but for FLASH a steady state exists only in the longitudinal direction.

Independent of the values of T1 and T2 and of the chosen imaging parameters, FISP can always be described by Eq. 1. Provided TR $\ll$ T2, a steady state will be obtained in both the transverse and the longitudinal direction, and in this case Eq. 1 for FISP can be simplified to Eq. 2 (*Weber* et al. 1986b):

$$I \sim \frac{\mathrm{rho} \cdot \sin\alpha \cdot \exp(-\,\mathrm{TE}/\mathrm{T2}^*)}{\mathrm{T1}/\mathrm{T2} + 1 - \cos\alpha \cdot (\mathrm{T1}/\mathrm{T2} - 1)} \,. \tag{2}$$

With FLASH, any steady state in the transverse direction is destroyed by the spoiler gradient. Therefore for FLASH Eq. 1 can be simplified to Eq. 3 (*Weber* et al. 1986b):

$$I \sim \frac{\mathrm{rho} \cdot (1 - \exp(-\,\mathrm{TR}/\mathrm{T1})) \cdot \sin\alpha \cdot \exp(-\,\mathrm{TE}/\mathrm{T2}^*)}{1 - \exp(-\,\mathrm{TR}/\mathrm{T1}) \cdot \cos\alpha} \,. \tag{3}$$

3 Analysis of Contrast Behaviour of FLASH and FISP

3.1 Approach

For FLASH and FISP a computer program was developed to calculate the signal intensity for any values of T1 and T2 and for different imaging parameters (TR, TE, flip angle α). The program was based on Eq. 1 for FISP[4] and Eq. 3 for FLASH. The signal intensities were calculated for different combinations of T1 (200 ms, 300 ms, ..., 1000 ms) and T2 (30 ms, 60 ms, 100 ms, 150 ms, 200 ms, 300 ms, 400 ms, ..., 1000 ms) simulating different kinds of tissues.

The imaging parameters were varied as follows:
- Flip angle α: 10°, 20°, 30°, 50°, 70°, 90°;
- TR: 30 ms, 100 ms, 200 ms, 500 ms;
- TE: 12 ms, 30 ms.

In order to assess the T1 or T2 weighting of the different pulse sequences, the signal intensities calculated for pulse sequences with varying imaging parameters, were plotted against T1 (for several representative constant T2 values) and against T2 (for several representative constant T1 values). From the slope of the resulting curves the influence of T1 or T2 on the signal intensity can be assessed:

---

[4] We have used Eq. 1, not Eq. 2, for FISP because the prerequisite TR $\ll T_2$, which has to be fulfilled before Eq. 1 can be replaced by Eq. 2, is not necessarily fulfilled for all tissues with different T2 values and for all settings of imaging parameters.

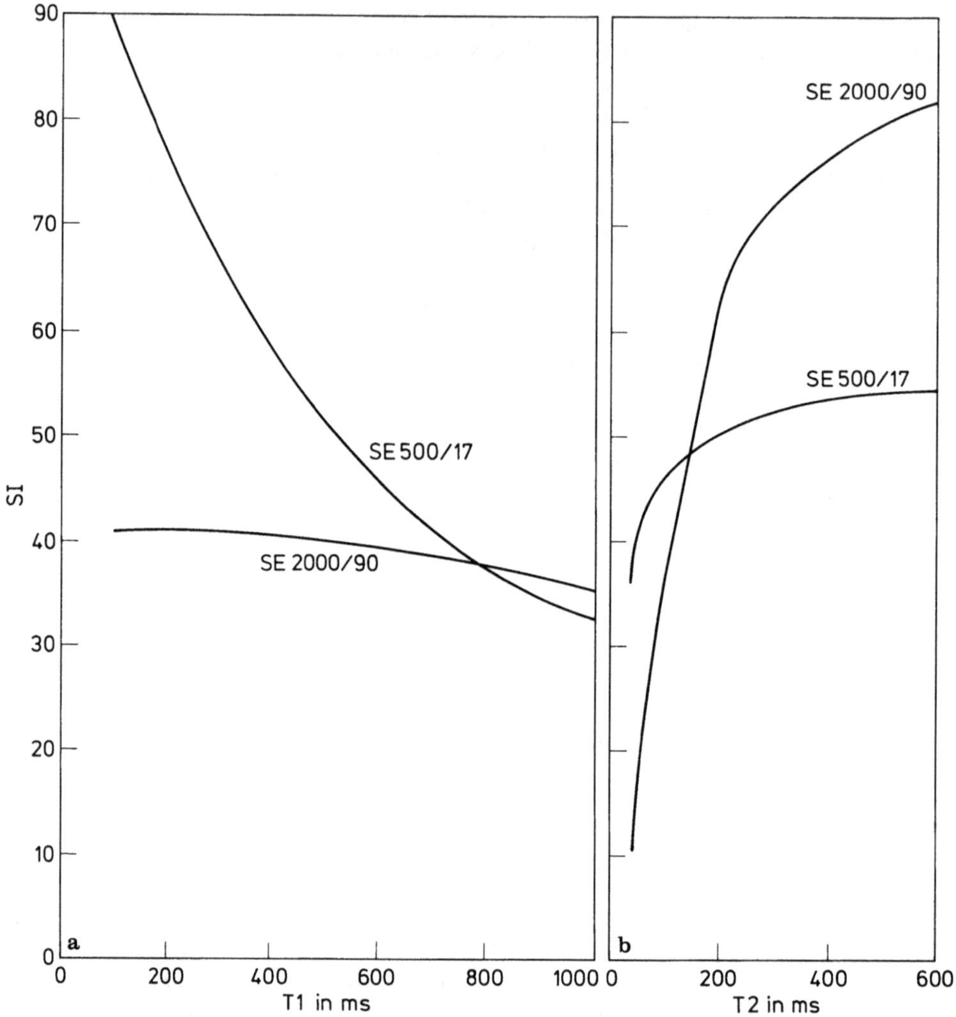

Fig. 2. a Influence of T1 on the signal intensity (SI) for T1-weighted (TR 500 ms, TE 17 ms) and T2-weighted (TR 2000 ms, TE 90 ms) SE sequences. T2 constant at 100 ms. **b** Influence of T2 on the SI for T1-weighted (TR 500 ms, TE 17 ms) and T2-weighted (TR 2000 ms, TE 90 ms) SE sequences. T1 constant at 600 ms

- The steeper the curve of the signal intensity depending on T1 (or T2), the stronger is the influence of T1 (or T2) on the signal intensity.
- Good T1 weighting exists when the signal intensity changes significantly with T1, but only slightly with T2. This is the case when the curve plotted against T1 is steep while the curce plotted against T2 is flat. An example of quite good T1 weighting (strong influence of T1 and little influence of T2 on the signal intensity) as can be achieved with SE: TR 500 ms, TE 17 ms is shown in Fig. 2a,b.

- Good T2 weighting exists, when the signal intensity changes significantly with T2 but only slightly or not at all with T1. Figure 2 also gives an example of strong T2 weighting, obtained by SE: TR 2000 ms, TE 90 ms.
- If neither T1 nor T2 influences the signal intensity significantly, the latter depends only on the proton density. Thus the pulse sequence is only proton densityweighted.

3.2 Analysis of FLASH with Various Flip Angles

Figure 3a, b illustrates the effect of T1 and T2 on the signal intensity of FLASH pulse sequences with varying flip angles (TR 30 ms, TE 12 ms). From these curves the following can be concluded:

- For flip angles of about 10° (and T2 > 100 ms) the effect of both T1 and T2 on the signal intensity is very small. Therefore the signal intensity is predominantly determined by the proton density.
- For flip angles of 30° - 90° the influence of T1 is increased, whereas the dependence of the signal intensity on T2 saturates when T2 is above 100 ms. For T2 values > 100 ms and Flip angles of 30° - 90° the influence of T2 on the signal intensity is little. Thus the influence of T1 will preponderate over that of T2, leading to quite good T1 weighting.

In summary, the following rules can be derived for FLASH (TR 30 ms, TE 12 ms) with varying flip angles: FLASH with a flip angle of about 10° is proton-density weighted. With flip angles between 30° and 90° the influence of T1 prevails, and quite good T1 weighting can be obtained provided T2 > 100 ms.

3.3 Analysis of FISP with Various Flip Angles

Figure 4a,b demonstrates the effect of T1 and T2 on the signal intensity of FISP with varying flip angles (TR 30 ms, TE 12 ms). From these curves the following can be derived:

- With flip angles of about 10° for FISP (as for FLASH) the influence of T1 and T2 is very small and these pulse sequences are therefore proton-density weighted.
- With increasing flip angles, up to 90°, the influence of both T1 and T2 increases significantly, as demonstrated by the increasing slopes of both curves. (Fig. 4a,b). Since, in contrast to FLASH (Fig. 3b), no saturation occurs, the influence of increasing T2 always counteracts the influence of increasing T1 and vice versa, resulting in a "mixed" pulse sequence.
- Only if T2 approaches T1 (i. e. with very long T2 values) is the relevant part of the curve which represents the T2 influence steeper than the relevant part of the curve which represents the T1 influence. This indicates a preponderant influence of T2. Therefore, when T2 approaches T1 (which is the case for ideal fluids), maximum signal intensity can be obtained with FISP and a Flip angle of 90°. This behaviour, different from that with FLASH, is caused by the transverse steady state and is therefore characteristic for FISP.

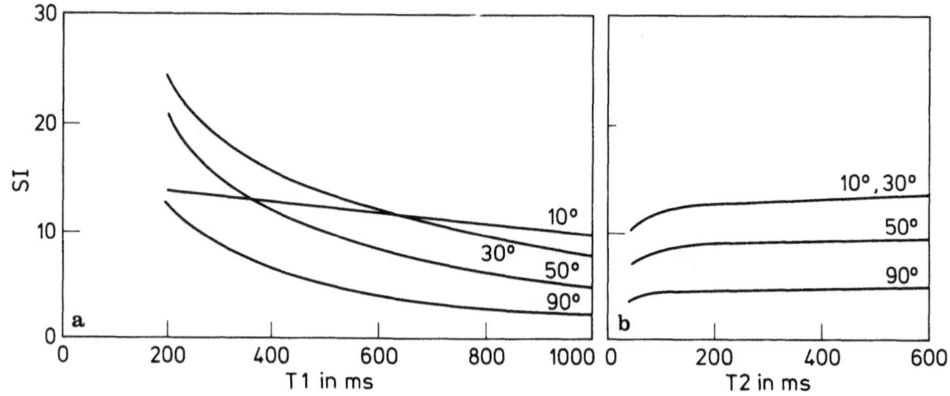

Fig. 3. a Influence of T1 on the signal intensity (SI) of FLASH sequences (TR 30 ms, TE 12 ms) with various flip angles (10°, 30°, 50°, 90°). T2 constant at 100 ms. **b** Influence of T2 on the SI of FLASH sequences (TR 30 ms, TE 12 ms) with various flip angles (10°, 30°, 50°, 90°). T1 constant at 600 ms

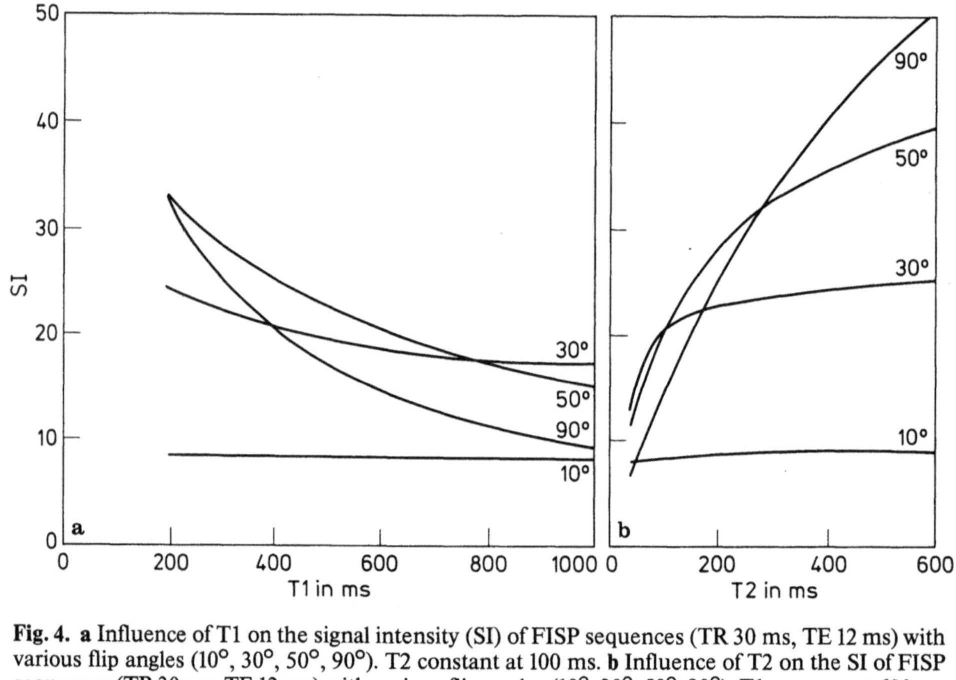

Fig. 4. a Influence of T1 on the signal intensity (SI) of FISP sequences (TR 30 ms, TE 12 ms) with various flip angles (10°, 30°, 50°, 90°). T2 constant at 100 ms. **b** Influence of T2 on the SI of FISP sequences (TR 30 ms, TE 12 ms) with various flip angles (10°, 30°, 50°, 90°). T1 constant at 600 ms

– The signal intensities with FISP are higher than with FLASH for most T1/T2 combinations, leading to a better signal-to-noise (S/N) ratio.

In summary, the following rules can be deduced for FISP with varying flip angles (TR 30 ms, TE 12 ms): With flip angles of about 10° FISP is proton-density weighted, like FLASH with a flip angle of 10°. With increasing flip angles the influence of both T1 and

T2 becomes strong. Only for ideal fluids (when T2 approaches T1), is a maximum signal intensity obtained, leading to high contrast.

One should not forget that the final image contrast between two tissues, A and B, will be determined not only by the relative T1 or T2 weighting of the chosen pulse sequence, but also, of course, by their T1 difference and their T2 difference. Therefore, in the individual case, the differences of both T1 and T2 in the tissues A and B will determine the necessary strength of T1 or T2 weighting for a good image contrast.

3.4 Influence of Echo Time

Variation of TE in FLASH and FISP sequences will have three different effects:

1. Depending on the TE of the gradient-echo sequence, the vectors of fat and water protons may point in the same direction (in-phase image), in different directions or in directly opposed directions (opposed-phase image). This effect has been described by *Dixon* (1984), who showed that using an in-phase and an opposed-phase image the signals of the fat and water protons can be separated. Figure 5 a, b shows examples of such in-phase and opposed-phase images, obtained with FLASH (TR 30 ms, TE 12 ms) at 1 T. Thus FISP or FLASH sequences with different TE can be used for fat-water separation (*Margosian* and *Deimling* 1986). However dealing with tissues which consist only of water protons, or with in-phase images only, this effect can be neglected if it is not desired.

2. Prolongation of TE will increase the effect of inhomogeneities: owing to the use of gradient echos in FLASH and FISP, magnetic field inhomogeneities are not compensated. The decay due to inhomogeneities plus the transverse relaxation is described by $T2^*$ and taken into account in Eqs. 1-3 by the factor $\exp(-TE/T2^*)$. Only for an absolutely homogeneous magnetic field is $T2^*$ equivalent to T2. For magnetic fields with inhomogeneities the term $\exp(-TE/T2^*)$ can be replaced in Eqs. 1-3 by

$$\exp(-TE/T2) \cdot \exp(-TE \cdot \gamma \cdot \Delta H_0/2) = \exp(-TE/T2) \cdot \text{const}$$

where γ = gyromagnetic constant, ΔH_0 = local inhomogeneity of the magnetic field[5]. The multiplication factor *const* describes the effects of local magnetic field inhomogeneities.

3. The effect of TE prolongation (from 12 to 30 ms) on the contrast behaviour of FLASH and FISP (for homogeneous magnets) has been studied by plotting the signal intensity against T1 and T2. In Fig. 6a-d the influence of T1 and T2 on the signal intensity can be assessed for TE of 12 ms and 30 ms and various FISP sequences (TR 100 ms, α 10°, 30°, 50°, 90°). From these curves the following can be derived:

- Only for FISP with $\alpha = 30°$ is the T2 influence improved for low T2 values (due to the increased slope of the left part of the curve in Fig. 5b). This will somewhat improve the overall T2 contrast for lower T2 values, considering that the influence of T1 does not increase further with prolongation of TE. Nevertheless, this pulse sequence still exhibits a mixed influence of T1 and T2.

[5] According to T. C. *Farrar* and E. D. *Becker* (1971), $(1/T2^*) = (1/T2) + (\gamma \cdot \Delta H_0/2)$.

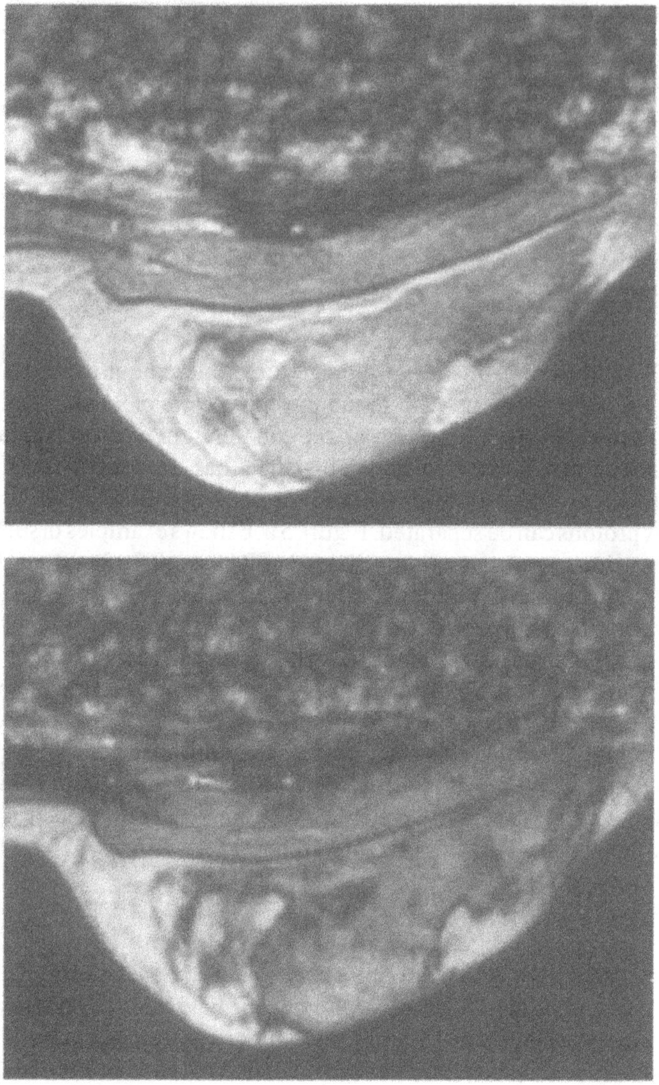

a

b

Fig. 5a, b. T1-weighted FLASH images (TR 40 ms, α 30°) of a normal breast at 1 T. **a** In-phase image at TE = 14 ms (two averages, imaging time 20 s). **b** Opposed-phase image at TE = 17 ms (two averages, imaging time 20 s). Owing to the fact that the vectors of fat and water subtract with opposed-phase pulse sequences, signal is zero in areas with similar amounts of fat and water protons. These areas are usually seen at the borders between fatty and glandular tissue and appear like frames

- For the other flip angles (50°, 90°) the contrast behaviour of FISP is not changed significantly (the resulting curves for TE = 12 ms and TE = 30 ms are almost parallel with similar slopes).

Figure 7a, b illustrates the influence of T1 and T2 on the signal intensity of FLASH (TR 100 ms, α 10°, 90°) for TE of 12 ms and 30 ms. For FLASH sequences the increase of

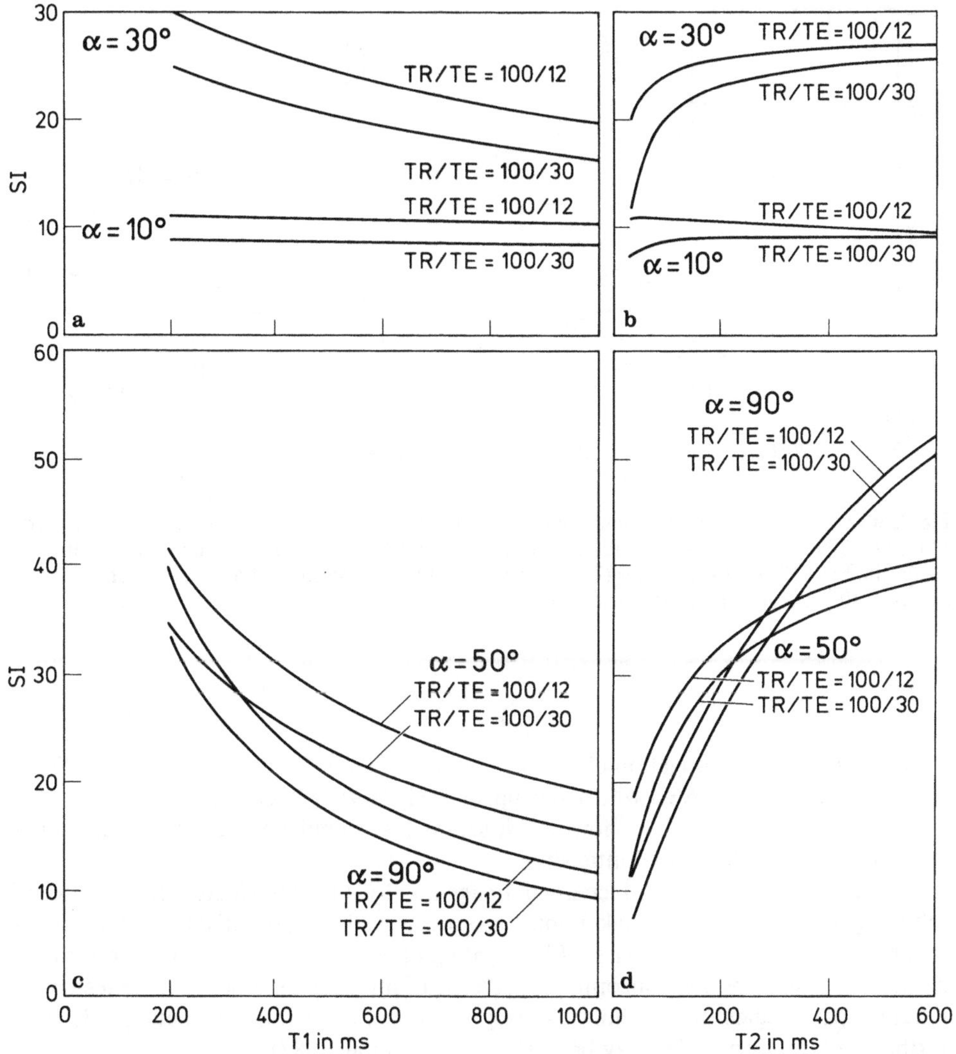

Fig. 6. a Influence of T1 on the signal intensity (SI) of FISP sequences (TR 100 ms) with TE of 12 ms and 30 ms at flip angles of 10° and 30°. T2 constant at 100 ms. **b** Influence of T2 on the SI of FISP sequences (TR 100 ms) with TE of 12 ms and 30 ms at flip angles of 10° and 30°. T1 constant at 600 ms. **c** Influence of T1 on the SI of FISP sequences (TR 100 ms) with TE of 12 ms and 30 ms at flip angles of 50° and 90°. T2 constant at 100 ms. **d** Influence of T2 on the SI of FISP sequences (TR 100 ms) with TE of 12 ms and 30 ms at flip angles of 50° and 90°. T1 constant at 600 ms

the T2 influence at lower T2 values could be observed with all flip angles (somewhat steeper left part of the curves plotted against T2). Since, however, FLASH sequences with flip angles of 30° - 90° are more T1 weighted, increased influence of T2 is undesirable. Only for FLASH sequences with a flip angle of 10° may the increased T2 contrast for lower flip angles be used, since here no counteracting effect of T1 is expected.

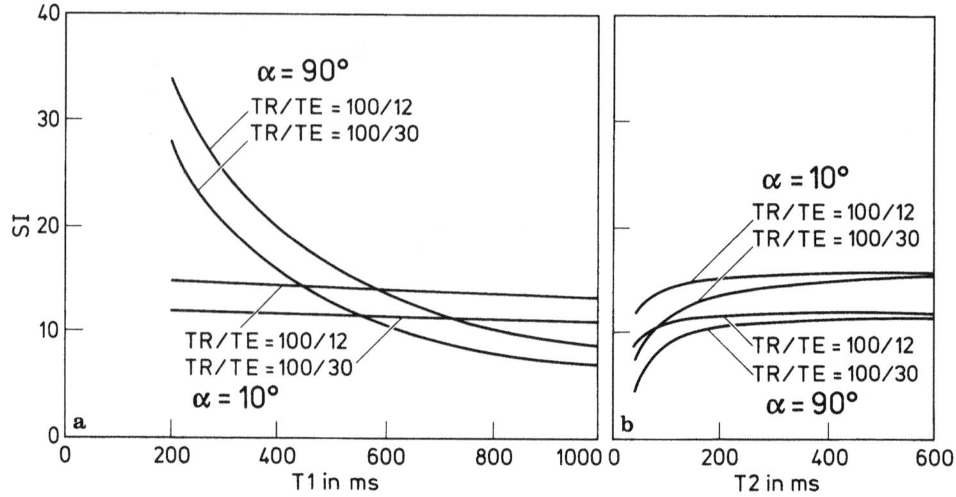

Fig. 7. a Influence of T1 on the signal intensity (SI) of FLASH sequences (TR 100 ms) with TE of 12 ms and 30 ms at representative flip angles of 10° and 90°. T2 constant at 100 ms. **b** Influence of T2 on the SI of FLASH sequences (TR 100 ms) with TE of 12 ms and 30 ms at representative flip angles of 10° and 90°. T1 constant at 600 ms

In conclusion, prolongation of TE does produce better T2 contrast for the relatively low T2 values when FLASH with a low flip angle (10°) is used. (A similar effect exists for FISP with a flip angle of 30°; however, it seems less significant due to the remaining influence of T1 on the signal intensity).

In reality, a simultaneous decrease of image quality due to the increased influence of inhomogeneities needs to be taken into account, as well as a potential fat-water separation effect. Whether the increased T2 weighting obtainable by TE prolongation will be sufficient considering the concomitant decrease of image quality needs to be tested for different pathologies in the clinical setting. With homogeneous magnetic fields even further prolongation of TE may be useful (*Buxton* et al. 1987).

3.5 Influence of Repetition Time

The effect of TR on the contrast obtainable by FISP and FLASH has been studied using computer analysis, with the following findings:

- With TR of up to 200 ms, the overall signal intensity for both FISP and FLASH increases. However, the general contrast behaviour of FLASH and FISP does not change significantly.
- With even greater prolongation of TR the steady state of FISP is progressively lost. Therefore the contrast behaviour of FISP will approach that of FLASH (i. e. the curve representing the influence of T2 will be flattened).

- The contrast behaviour of FLASH with a flip angle of 90° will finally resemble the contrast behaviour of SE sequences with the same parameters.

In summary, the prolongation of TR to 200 ms will improve the S/N ratio but simultaneously increase the imaging time. The overall contrast behaviour does not change significantly. Whether further increase of TR above 200 ms will provide significant advantages needs to be shown, considering the prolonged imaging time.

3.6 Choice of Appropriate Pulse Sequence

FLASH and FISP pulse sequences are pulse sequences with a mixed counteracting effect of T1 and T2 on the signal intensity. Therefore the contrast between normal tissues and those abnormal tissues in which both T1 and T2 are prolonged may be slight. In order to avoid this problem and to improve this contrast, it is necessary to find the best possible T1 or T2 weighting.

Table 1 gives an overview of the pulse sequences which promise the best possible T1, T2 or proton-density weighting according to the above calculations. With these pulse sequences acceptable T1 weighting and good proton-density weighting can be obtained. No pulse sequence with a genuinely good T2 weighting (and little influence of T1 on the signal intensity) could be found using TE values below 30 ms. Therefore it will be necessary to check critically for which pathological lesions the obtainable contrast will suffice. With further prolongation of TE, improved T2 weighting may be expected, but a concomitant decrease of image quality must be taken into account.

Table 1. An overview of pulse sequences which appear to provide the best possible T1, T2 or proton-density weighting

Pulse sequence	Flip angle	TR (ms)	TE (ms)	Weighting	Range of optimum T1, T2 or proton-density contrast
FLASH	10°	30	12	Proton density	Any T1 or T2 values
FLASH	>50°	30	12	T1	T2 above 100 ms
FLASH	10°	100[a]	>30	T2	Low T2 (compared with T1)
FISP	90°	30	12	T2	T2 approaching T1 (i. e. relatively high T2)

[a] TR needs to be higher than TE. The relatively high TR has no significant influence on the contrast, but improves the S/N ratio

3.7 Phantom Measurements

In addition to merely theoretical evaluation of the contrast behaviour of FLASH and FISP sequences, these sequences were also analysed using a total of 25 phantoms consisting of gels with different T1 and T2 values (*Schultz* and *Lutz* 1986). These phantoms were measured with various FLASH and FISP pulse sequences (α 10°, 30°, 50°, 70°, 90°; TE 12 ms, 22 ms; TR 30 ms, 100 ms, 300 ms) using a MAGNETOM (Siemens) at 1 T. The first results of these measurements have been reported previously (*Heywang* et al. 1987): It could be shown that, in general, good qualitative agreement existed between the theoretical calculations and the phantom measurements, leading to the same conclusions. In order better to check the quantitative correlation, a more exact phantom is being developed.

4 Clinical Examples

The first clinical applications of FLASH and FISP have yielded results agreeing well with the theoretical results. Some other factors influencing the image contrast in clinical examinations will be mentioned briefly.

Figure 8a - d shows representative FLASH and FISP images of a normal brain, proving that quite good T1 weighting, some T2 weighting and good proton-density weighting can be obtained. SE sequences with good T1, T2 and proton-density weighting are shown in Fig. 8e - g for comparison.

Figure 9a - f shows a plaque of multiple sclerosis imaged using SE and fast-imaging pulse sequences. This example shows that the visualization of pathology by the T2-weighted fast-imaging pulse sequences has frequently been inferior to the information provided by the corresponding SE sequences. Similar experience has also been reported by other authors and for other organs, like liver or breast (*Friedmann* et al. 1987; *Kaiser* and *Oppelt* 1987; *Weiss* et al. 1987). According to our early experience, improvements of the T2 weighting can, however, be expected when TE is prolonged and more acquisitions are used. For this purpose a new FLASH multi-echo sequence will be tested.

Until more clinical experience has been gathered, fast-imaging sequences cannot be regarded as reliable in those cases where good T2 contrast is diagnostically important.

In combination with paramagnetic contrast agents the results were in general significantly better (*Heywang* et al. 1987; *Kaiser* and *Oppelt* 1987; *Laniado* et al. 1986; *Karis* et al. 1986). This can be explained by the fact that gadolinium-DTPA (Gd-DTPA) shortens T1 significantly, but T2 only slightly. Owing to the high sensitivity of fast-imaging sequences to small amounts of paramagnetic contrast medium, and to the short imaging time, they appear especially suitable for dynamic contrast studies (*Laniado* et al. 1986; *Karis* et al. 1986). Figure 10 shows a dynamic contrast study of a Gd-DTPA-enhanced breast carcinoma.

For contrast studies, T1-weighted FLASH sequences with pulse angles of 30°-90° have proved quite good. Unless 3D imaging was employed, we used flip angles of 30°-50° because of their good T1 weighting and the absence of an M-shaped slice profile, which appears at higher flip angles (*Frahm* et al. 1987; *Harms* 1986).

The use of FISP with high flip angles (90°) may be advantageous in those cases where good contrast between liquids and solid tissues is desirable, e.g. for the evaluation of joints (*König* et al. 1986). Figure 11 shows a FISP image, with 90° flip angle, of a normal knee with high contrast between joint fluid, cartilage and menisci.

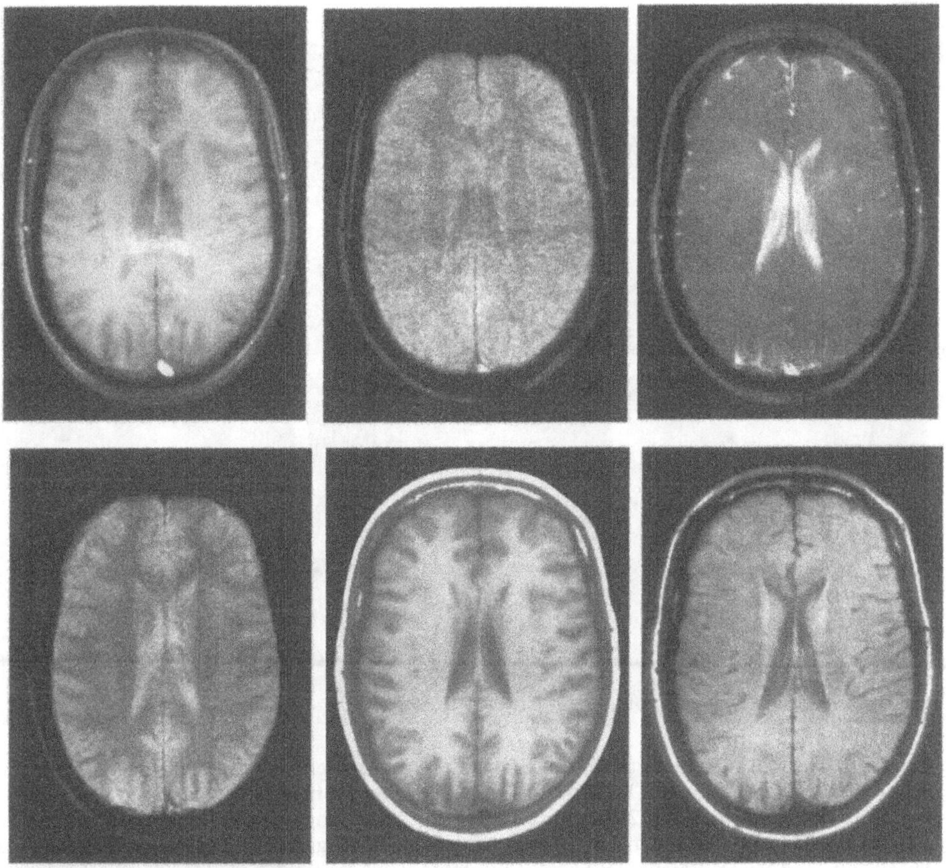

a b c

d e f

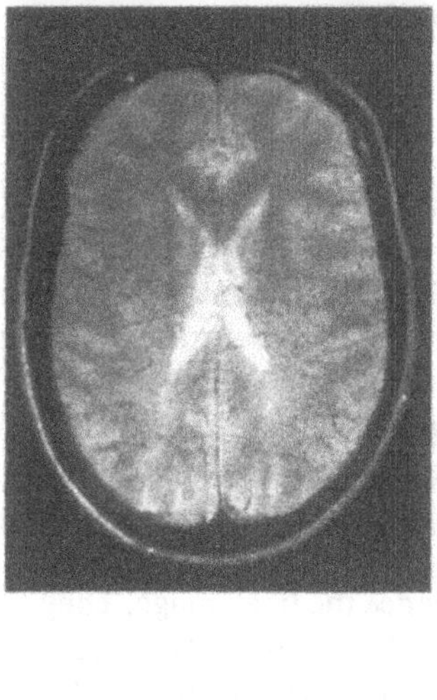

g

Fig. 8a–g. Representative slice of a normal brain at the level of the ventricles imaged with different pulse sequences. **a** FLASH (α 50°, TR 30 ms, TE 12 ms); T1 weighted; two averages; imaging time per slice 15 s. **b** FLASH (α 10°, TR 30 ms, TE 12 ms); proton-density weighted; two averages; imaging time per slice 15 s. **c** FISP (α 90°, TR 30 ms, TE 12 ms); mixed pulse sequence; two averages; imaging time per slice 15 s. **d** FLASH (α 10°, TR 100 ms, TE 30 ms); somewhat T2 weighted; two averages; imaging time per slice 51 s. **e** SE TR 500 ms, TE 17 ms; T1 weighted; two averages. **f** SE TR 2000 ms, TE 28 ms; proton-density weighted; one average. **g** SE TR 2000 ms, TE 90 ms; T2 weighted; one average

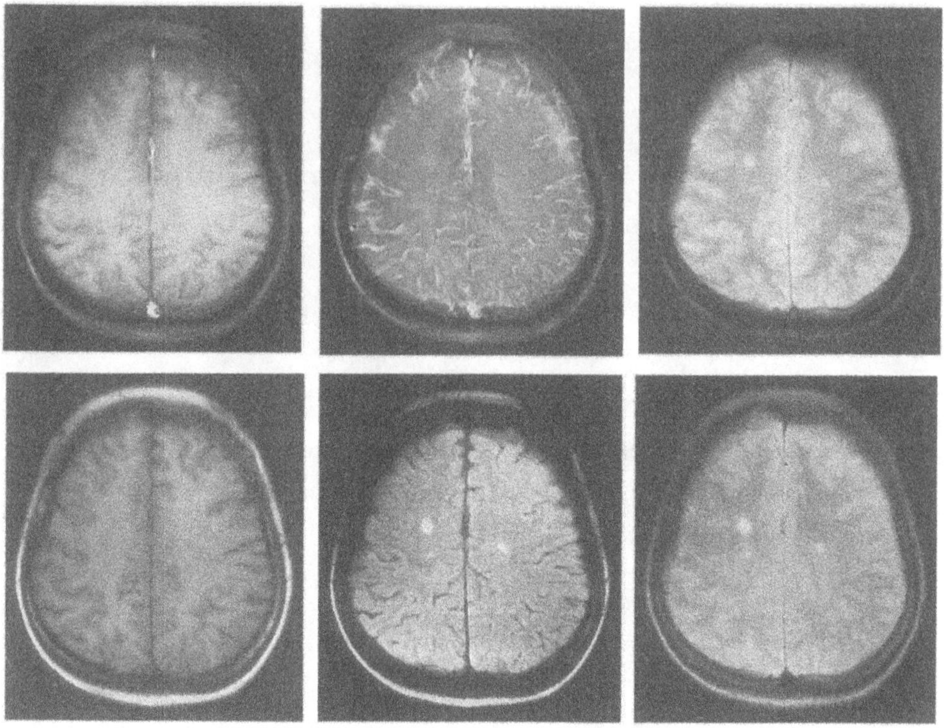

Fig. 9a–f. Slice through the brain in a patient with multiple sclerosis. Several plaques are present. **a** FLASH (α 50°, TR 30 ms, TE 12 ms); T1 weighted; four averages; imaging time per slice 30 s. **b** FISP (α 90°, TR 30 ms, TE 12 ms); mixed pulse sequence; four averages; imaging time per slice 30 s. **c** FLASH (α 10°, TR 100 ms, TE 30 ms); somewhat T2 weighted; four averages; imaging time per slice 100 s. **d** SE TR 500 ms, TE 17 ms; T1 weighted; two averages. **e** SE TR 2000 ms, TE 28 ms; proton-density weighted; one average. **f** SE TR 2000 ms, TE 90 ms; T2 weighted; one average

When exploiting the interesting new possibilities of fast-imaging sequences – like 3D imaging within acceptable imaging time and thin slices, dynamic contrast studies or even dynamic studies of heart motion or blood flow (*Axel* et al. 1986; *Rienmüller* 1987; *Higgins* 1987; *Utz* et al. 1986) – the disadvantages arising from their different contrast behaviour and from changes in susceptibility must be considered. The problems relating to the contrast theoretically achievable with these mixed pulse sequences have been discussed above. Whereas the influence of the imaging parameters on the contrast can be calculated, the influence of changes in susceptibility is difficult to assess in clinical examinations and needs further investigation.

Artefacts due to changes of the susceptibility also influence the final image. They are caused by adjacent bone or air and are thus encountered close to the sinuses or bony skull, as shown in Fig. 12, or in the neighbourhood of bowel loops in the liver or abdomen (*Oppelt* et al. 1986; *Buxton* et al. 1987; *Heywang* et al. 1987). Metal clips, which also cause changes in susceptibility, produce more prominent artefacts with FLASH or FISP than with SE sequences, as demonstrated in Fig. 13.

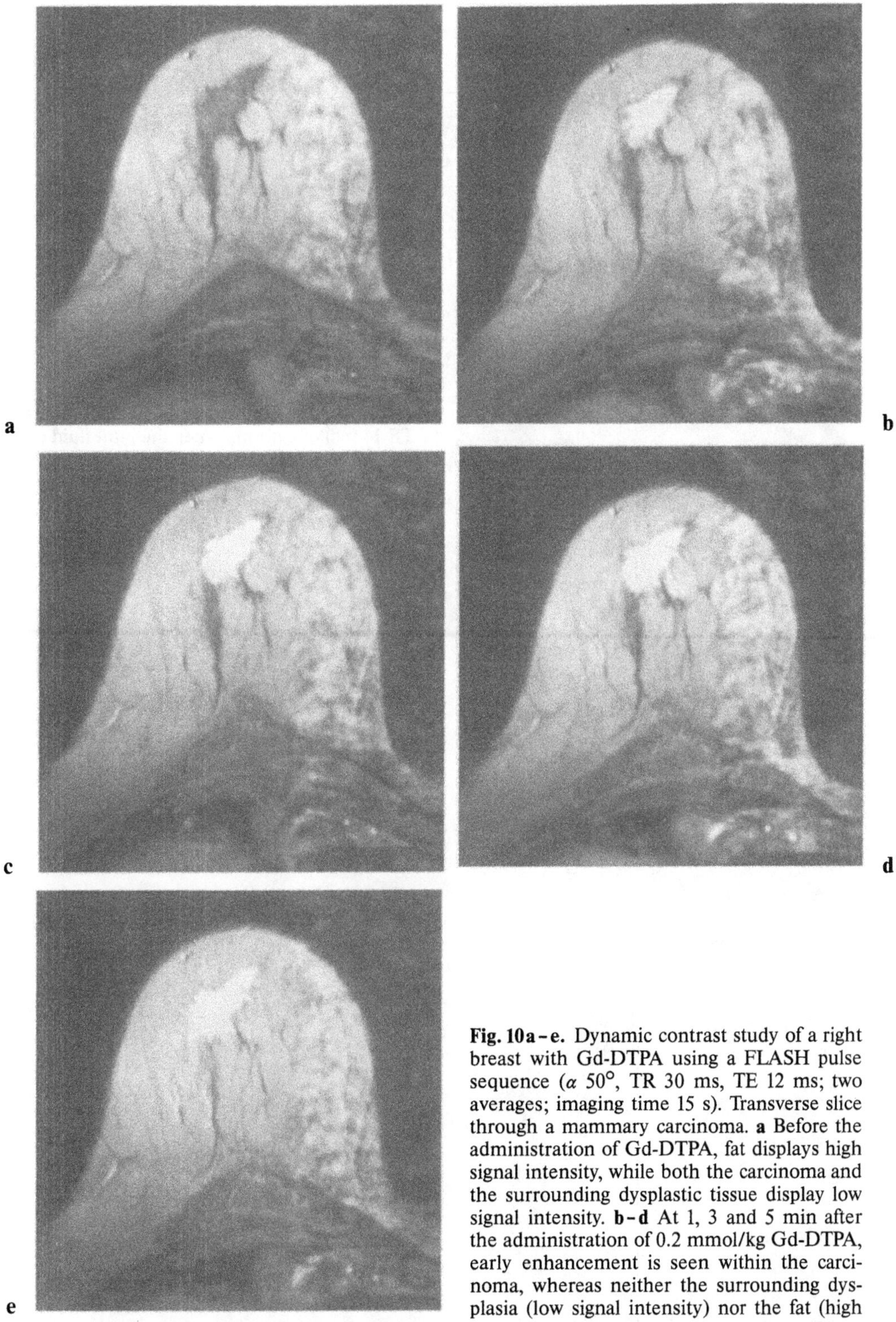

Fig. 10a–e. Dynamic contrast study of a right breast with Gd-DTPA using a FLASH pulse sequence (*α* 50°, TR 30 ms, TE 12 ms; two averages; imaging time 15 s). Transverse slice through a mammary carcinoma. **a** Before the administration of Gd-DTPA, fat displays high signal intensity, while both the carcinoma and the surrounding dysplastic tissue display low signal intensity. **b–d** At 1, 3 and 5 min after the administration of 0.2 mmol/kg Gd-DTPA, early enhancement is seen within the carcinoma, whereas neither the surrounding dysplasia (low signal intensity) nor the fat (high signal intensity) exhibit a significant increase. **e** At 15 min after the administration of Gd-DTPA strong enhancement is again seen within the carcinoma. Slight enhancement ist now also noted within the dysplastic tissue

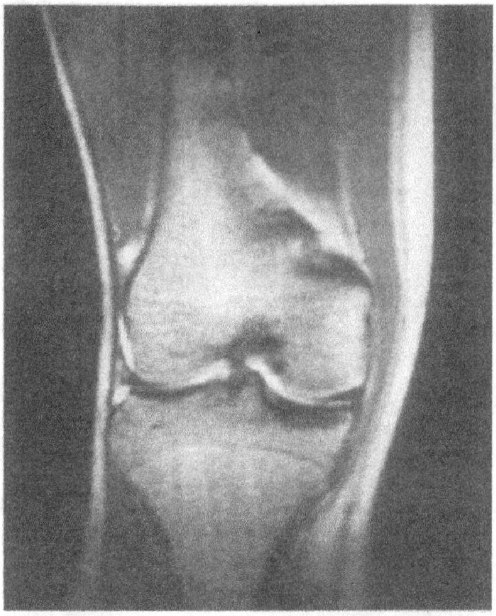

Fig. 11. In this FISP image (α 90°, TR 40 ms, TE 14 ms) of a normal knee the joint fluid exhibits high signal intensity, in contrast to the low signal intensity of the menisci and ligaments. (two averages; imaging time 20 s)

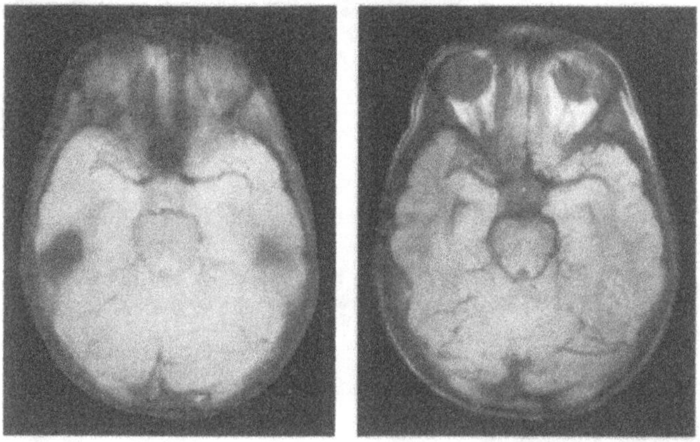

a b

Fig. 12a, b. A slice of the brain above the petrous bones. **a** SE TR 2000 ms, TE 28 ms. **b** FLASH (α 10°, TR 30 ms, TE 12 ms). The nearby petrous bones cause significant artefacts (loss of signal intensity) with this pulse sequence owing to changes of susceptibility

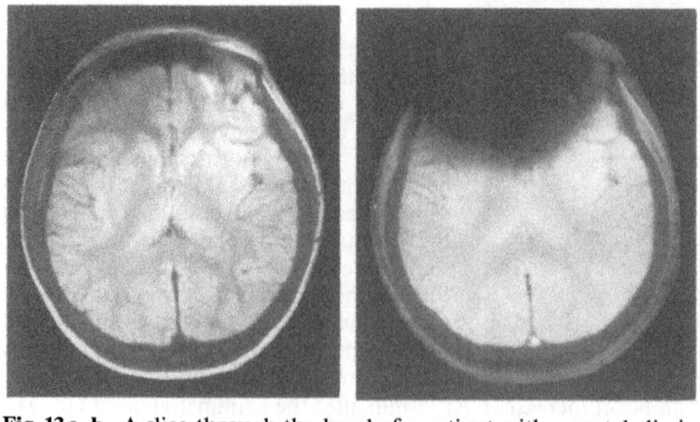

a b

Fig. 13a, b. A slice through the head of a patient with a metal clip in the skull. **a** SE TR 2000 ms, TE 28 ms. **b** FLASH (α 10°, TR 30 ms, TE 12 ms). Artefact (loss of signal intensity) owing to the metal clip significantly more marked with the fast-imaging sequence

5 Conclusions

It has been shown that by varying the imaging parameters, images can be obtained with either good proton-density weighting, an acceptable T1 weighting or some T2 weighting. Excellent contrast between liquids and solid tissues is obtained by FISP with a flip angle of 90°. However, due to the counteracting influences of both T1 and T2 on the signal intensity, which is characteristic especially for FISP, some solid lesions may show only slight or insufficient contrast. Improvement of the T2 weighting with the concomitant decrease in S/N ratio by increased prolongation of TE requires further clinical testing. It is essential to find out, for which tissues or lesions the obtainable T1 or T2 weighting and the image quality will be sufficient. Further research with 3D and dynamic imaging of the breast with contrast medium is now confirming the here shown advantages of fast imaging sequences for MRI with paramagnetic contrast agent.

In exploiting the potential advantages of FLASH and FISP sequences, the influence of the imaging parameters, of $T2^*$, of susceptibility and of artefacts of susceptibility and motion on final image contrast and on image quality must be considered.

References

Axel L, Reichek N, Schiebler M et al. (1986) Rapid small flip angle MRI: valvular insufficiency. Radiology 161 (P): 338

Buxton RB, Edelman RR, Rosen BR et al. (1987) Contrast in rapid MR imaging: T1- and T2-weighted imaging. J Com. Assist Tomogr 11 (1): 7 - 15

Dixon WT (1984) Simple proton spectroscopic imaging. Radiology 153 (1): 189 - 194

Farrar TC, Becker EJ (1971) Pulse and Fourier transform NMR. Academic New York

Frahm J, Haase A, Matthaei D (1986) Rapid NMR imaging of dynamic processes using the FLASH technique. Magn Reson Med 3: 321 - 327

Frahm J, Merboldt KD, Hänicke W (1987) Neue Ergebnisse mit der FLASH-Tomographie. In: Lissner J, Doppman JL, Margulis AR (eds) MR'87. Schnetztor Verlag, Konstanz, 21 - 24

Friedmann G, Krestin G, Bunke J (1987) Kontraste an normalen und pathologischen Geweben - Gegenüberstellung Spinecho und FFE-Verfahren. In: Lissner J, Doppman JR, Margulis A (eds) MR'87. Schnetztor Verlag, Konstanz, 30 - 34

Harms, SE (1986) Fast imaging schemes and 3-dimensional image acquisitions. Radiology 161 (P): 77

Heywang SH, Köbrunner G, Wolf A et al. (1987) Klinische Anwendung von Fast Imaging-Techniken. In: Lissner J, Doppman JL, Margulis A (eds) MR 87 Referateband. Schnetztor, pp 35-38

Higgins CB (1987) EKG-gated cine MRI of the heart: anatomy and function. In: Lissner J, Doppman JL, Margulis A (1987) MR 87, Referateband. Schnetztor, (inpress)

Kaiser WA, Oppelt A (1987) KST der Mamma mit Schnellbildverfahren. In: Lissner J, Doppman JL, Margulis A (eds) MR 87, Referateband. Schnetztor, pp 303-310

Karis, JP, Fram EK, Johnson GA et al. (1986) Contrast-dependence in limited-angle MR imaging. Radiology 161 (P): 68

König H, Sauter R, Kueper K et al. (1986) MRI of articular cartilage disorders: specificity of fast imaging and CHESS. Radiology 161 (P): 312

Krestin GP, Friedmann G, Promper CH et al. (1986) Experimental MR studies with fast imaging sequences (FFE) at 1.5 T: signal contrast in normal and pathological tissues. Radiology 161 (P): 333

Laniado M, Kornmesser W, Deimling M, Felix R (1986) Dynamic MR imaging of renal tumors: fast imaging and Gd-DTPA. Radiology 161 (P): 119

Mansfield P, Morris PG (1982) NMR imaging in biomedicine, suppl 2. In: Waugh JS (ed.) Advances in magnetic resonance. Academic, New York, pp 75 - 77

Margosian P, Deimling M (1986) Clinical tests of chemical shift imaging using fast gradient echoes. Radiology 161 (P): 211

Matthaei D, Frahm J, Haase A et al. (1986) Möglichkeiten der schnellen Kernspintomographie mit dem FLASH-Verfahren. Zentralbl Radiologie 132 (5): 358

Mills TC, Ortendahl DA, Hylton NM et al. (1987) Partial flip angle MR imaging. Radiology 162: 531 - 539

Oppelt A, Gaumann R, Barfuß H et al. (1986) FISP: eine neue schnelle Pulssequenz für die Kernspintomographie. Electromed (EnglEd) 54: 15 - 17

Rienmüller R, Brunnhölzl W, Gärtner CH et al (1987) MR bei transplantierten Herzen. In: Lissner J, Doppman JR, Margulis A (eds) MR'87. Schnetztor Verlag, Konstanz 69 - 77

Schultz E, Lutz NW (1986) Gewebeäquivalente MRI-Phantommaterialien - Eigenschaften und Anwendungsmöglichkeiten. Zentralbl Radiologie 132 (5): 376

Utz JA, Herfkens R, Glover GH (1986) Dynamic MRI of the heart. Radiology 161 (P): 185

Weber H, Deimling M (1987) Schnelle Bildgebung mit FISP und FLASH. Vergleich des Kontrastverhaltens und Anwendungsmöglichkeiten. In: Lissner J, Doppman JL, Margulis A (eds) MR'87, Referateband, Schnetztor (inpress)

Weber H, Purdy D, Deimling M, Oppelt A (1986a) Contrast behaviour of FLASH and FISP: results from synthetic images. Radiology 161 (P): 67

Weber H, Purdy D, Deimling M, Oppelt A (1986b) Contrast behaviour of the fast imaging sequences FLASH and FISP: results from synthetic images. Book of abstracts vol 3. Society of Magnetic Resonance in Medicine Berkeley, CA 94704, USA 957

Weiss T, Mitsch E, Laniado M et al. (1987) Schnelle Kernspintomographie. RD 1 FO 146 (2): 214 - 222

Ultrasound of the Hip Joint: Experimental and Clinical Studies

R. Langer[1]

[1] Radiologische Klinik und Poliklinik (Dir.: Prof. Dr. R. Felix), Freie Universität Berlin, Klinikum Rudolf Virchow - Charlottenburg, Spandauer Damm 130, D-1000 Berlin 19

1 Introduction

Congenital hip dysplasia and dislocation are common diseases of newborns and small infants, with frequently severe consequences if orthopaedic therapy is not initiated at an early stage. Therefore many clinicians have been looking for a simple method for the investigation of the hip joint in the early neonatal period.

Up to 1980 the diagnosis of hip dysplasia could usually not be made before the 3rd month of life, by means of pelvic roentgenography. Only incomplete or complete unilateral dislocations were diagnosed in the neonatal age group. In 1980, however, *Graf*, an Austrian orthopaedic surgeon, began using ultrasound investigation of the hip joint in newborns and small infants in order to make an early diagnosis and to avoid radiation exposure.

The intention of the present study was to compare ultrasound of the hip joint with other established diagnostic procedures and to establish whether it is suitable as a screening procedure in newborns.

2 Incidence of Congenital Hip Dysplasia and Dislocation

In 1972 *Barlow* reported that 90 % of hips which are unstable at birth develop to normal joints spontaneously without any therapy. *Visser* (1984) thus suggested determining the percentage of hip dislocations after the 2nd - 3rd month of life so that children with spontaneous stabilisation would be excluded.

The reported incidence of dislocating hips in newborns differs from 1.7 ‰ to 17 ‰ (*Barlow* 1962; *Lefaure* et al. 1985; *Mitchell* 1972; *Palmen* 1984; *Rosen* 1962; *Tredwell* and *Bell* 1981; *Visser* 1984). In Europe there are geographical differences in the incidence of congenital hip dysplasia. In Central Europe the incidence is about 1 ‰ - 2 ‰ (*Dunn* 1969, 1974; *Haike* 1965).

For Germany, *Gladel* (1983) reported a 2 ‰ - 5 ‰ incidence of unstable hips in all newborns; he observed one complete dislocation in 100 unstable hips. *Palmen* (1984) reported a 6.2 ‰ incidence of incomplete dislocations in Sweden. He had examined 28 000 newborns clinically from 1950 to 1974. A high incidence of congenital hip dysplasia and dislocation is well known in parts of Yugoslavia and Czechoslovakia.

The male to female ratio is 1 : 4. Left hips are affected twice as often as right hips.

3 Familial Disposition of Congenital Hip Dysplasia

In 1970 *Wynne-Davies* described the existence of a familial disposition towards congenital hip dysplasia. If siblings suffer from hip dysplasia, the risk increases to 6 %. If one of the parents is affected the risk for a neonate rises to 12 %, and if both a parent and a sibling suffer from hip dysplasia, the risk for each further child becomes 36 %.

4 Diagnostic Procedures for Congenital Hip Dysplasia and Dislocation

Congenital hip dysplasia must be diagnosed early if the best therapeutic results are to be achieved (*Bayer* 1958; *Becker* 1963; *Dörr* 1966; *Frischknecht* 1957; *Haike* 1965; *Palmen* 1984; *Tönnis* 1980). If the diagnosis is made soon after birth, complete recovery is possible in nearly all cases; if therapy starts after the 4th month of life, complete recovery can be achieved in only two-thirds of the patients (*Graf* 1985; *Graf* and *Schuler* 1986; *Tönnis* 1976, 1980). Swedish specialists have accumulated great experience in clinical examination. A total of 28 000 newborns were investigated between 1950 and 1974 by *Palmen* (1984).

In France a radiological screening programme in the 3rd to 4th month of life was still being discussed in 1985 in spite of the possibility of hip ultrasound (*Lefaure* et al. 1985).

The following clinical and radiological diagnostic methods were used to diagnose hip dysplasia before the introduction of ultrasound of the hip, or are additional diagnostic techniques: history, visual inspection, clinical examination, plain X-ray studies of the pelvis (beyond the neonatal age group), arthrography, computed tomography and magnetic resonance imaging.

4.1 History

An increased incidence of hip joint dysplasia and dislocation in cases of familial disposition has been proved by clinical studies (*Palmen* 1984; *Visser* 1984; *Wynne-Davies* 1970). Therefore it is necessary to ask the parents if a familial disposition is present.

The course of the pregnancy is also an important factor. It has been reported in several publications (*Dunn* 1969, 1974; *Faber* 1938; *Palmen* 1984; *Rosen* 1962; *Visser* 1984) that breech or transverse presentation, twins and oligohydramnios are predisposing factors for hip dysplasia because of the reduced intrauterine movement of the legs.

4.2 Visual Inspection

Clubfoot and other foot abnormalities are often combined with hip dysplasia and dislocation (*Graf* 1985, 1986; *Palmen* 1984; *Sinios* 1969; *Visser* 1984).

External rotation of the upper leg, reduced mobility of a leg, and difference in leg length may result from hip dysplasia. In a small proportion of patients, asymmetrical gluteal folds coincide with hip dysplasia. Many publications, however, habe shown that the diagnostic value of such folds is low (*Graf* 1983a, b, 1985; *Graf* and *Schuler* 1986; *Hellige* 1986; *Langer* 1987; *Langer* and *Kaufmann* 1986; *Schulz* et al. 1986); they mostly result from a curved position of the newborn during visual inspection.

4.3 Clinical Examination

Barlow's and Ortolani's signs may be present in newborns up to 1 week old with unstable hips (*Barlow* 1962; *Palmen* 1984; *Rosen* 1962) but after the 2nd week of life these signs are no longer evident. With an unstable hip the femoral head can first be dislocated outside the acetabulum and later repositioned into the acetabulum on abduction of the upper leg. After the 1st week of life the abduction of the hip joints should be tested (*Mitchell* 1972; *Palmen* 1984; *Rosen* 1962).

Abduction of 80° - 90° from the midline in newborns and 60° - 75° in the 2nd and 3rd months of life is physiological. If abduction is reduced to less than 45° from the midline, hip dysplasia or dislocation is usally present. If it is reduced to 45° - 60°, "limited abduction" can be diagnosed and hip dysplasia must be suspected (*Mitchell* 1972; *Palmen* 1984; *Rosen* 1962; *Schuster* 1968). The abduction test must not be performed in babies with general muscular hypertonia.

4.4 Plain X-Ray Surveys of the Pelvis

Up to the 3rd month of life, pelvic roentgenography is of no value for the diagnosis of hip dysplasia (*Graf* 1980, 1983a, b, 1985; *Graf* and *Schuler* 1986; *Imhäuser* 1982; *Tönnis* and *Brunken* 1968). The cartilaginous femoral head and acetabular rim cannot be visualized by X-ray studies; only the ossified parts of the hip joints are seen. Plain X-ray surveys of the pelvis were usually performed after the 3rd month of life before the introduction of ultrasound of the hip.

4.5 Arthrography

The advantage of arthrography is the visualization of the cartilaginous parts of the hip joint (*Graf* 1985; *Izadpanah* 1979; *Newberg* et al. 1985; *Schwetlik* and *Kasparek* 1969; *Strife* et al. 1984; *Thomas* 1960; *Tönnis* 1980).

There are three established techniques of hip arthrography:

1. Arthrography with positive iodine-containing contrast medium
2. Arthrography with negative contrast medium (air)
3. Double-contrast arthrography, a combination of techniques 1 and 2

The most important advantage of hip arthrography was demonstrated by *Faber* (1938), who showed by means of arthrography that parts of the cartilaginous acetabulum can be dislocated into the joint in cases of hip dislocations. Hip arthrography is, however, an invasive diagnostic procedure with a certain risk of infection (*Newberg* et al. 1985).

4.6 Computed Tomography

The usefulness of computed tomography (CT) for the diagnosis of hip dysplasia or dislocation is limited because of the axial nature of the tomograms. The collodiaphyseal angle, as well as dislocation of the hip joint, may be only partly demonstrated; in some cases reconstructed coronal slices are necessary. An advantage of CT is the direct visualization of the cartilaginous parts of the femoral head and the acetabulum as well as of the soft tissues of the hip joint.

Complete dislocation of the joint can be diagnosed by CT, but a slight lateralization may escape diagnosis. Another disadvantage of CT is the requirement for a fixed position of the hip joints throughout the examination, which mostly necessitates heavy sedation or general anaesthesia.

4.7 Magnetic Resonance Imaging

Magnetic resonance imaging (MRI) in newborns is also limited by the necessity of immobilization during the examination. Single cases of incomplete or complete dislocation of the hip have been demonstrated by *Moore* et al. (1985). Two advantages of MRI are the possibility of examining infants in a cast and its capacity for multiplanar axial, sagittal and coronal slices.

In summary, CT and MRI are not routine methods for the diagnosis of congenital hip dislocation, but reserved for single patients with special problems.

5 Ultrasound of the Hip

In 1980 *Graf* published a preliminary report of the ultrasound investigation of the hip joints of newborns. The major advantage of the method is its direct visualization of the cartilaginous parts of the joint and the soft tissues, whereas on plain X-rays only the ossified parts of the joint are seen.

The first classification of hip joint ultrasonography was established by Graf. Initially he described four types of hip dysplasia and dislocation (Fig. 1); later, more and more subdivisions were introduced. The types are defined morphologically by measurement of two angles, α and β. This requires the drawing of three lines on the ultrasound picture. At present the following types of hip joint are defined (Table 1):

Table 1. Grafs extended classification of ultrasound findings in the hip of newborns

Type	Bony edge	Cartilaginous edge	α	β	Position of femoral epiphysis	Age (months)
Ia	Angled	Anechoic/sharp	>60°	<55°	Centered	0-12
Ib	Angled	Anechoic/broad	>60°	55°-70°	Centered	0-12
IIa	Rounded	Anechoic/broad	50°-60°	55°-70°	Centered	0- 3
IIb	Rounded	Anechoic/broad	43°-60°	55°-77°	Centered	3-12
IIc	Rounded/flat	Anechoic/broad	43°-50°	55°-77°	Centered (→ lateralization)	0-12
D	Rounded/flat	Anechoic/broad	43°-50°	>77°	Lateralized	0-12
IIIa	Flat	Anechoic/broad	<43°	>77°	Dislocated	0-12
IIIb	Flat	Echoic/broad	<43°	>77°	Dislocated	0-12
IV	Flat	Anechoic/echoic	<43°	Measurement impossible	Dislocated	0-12

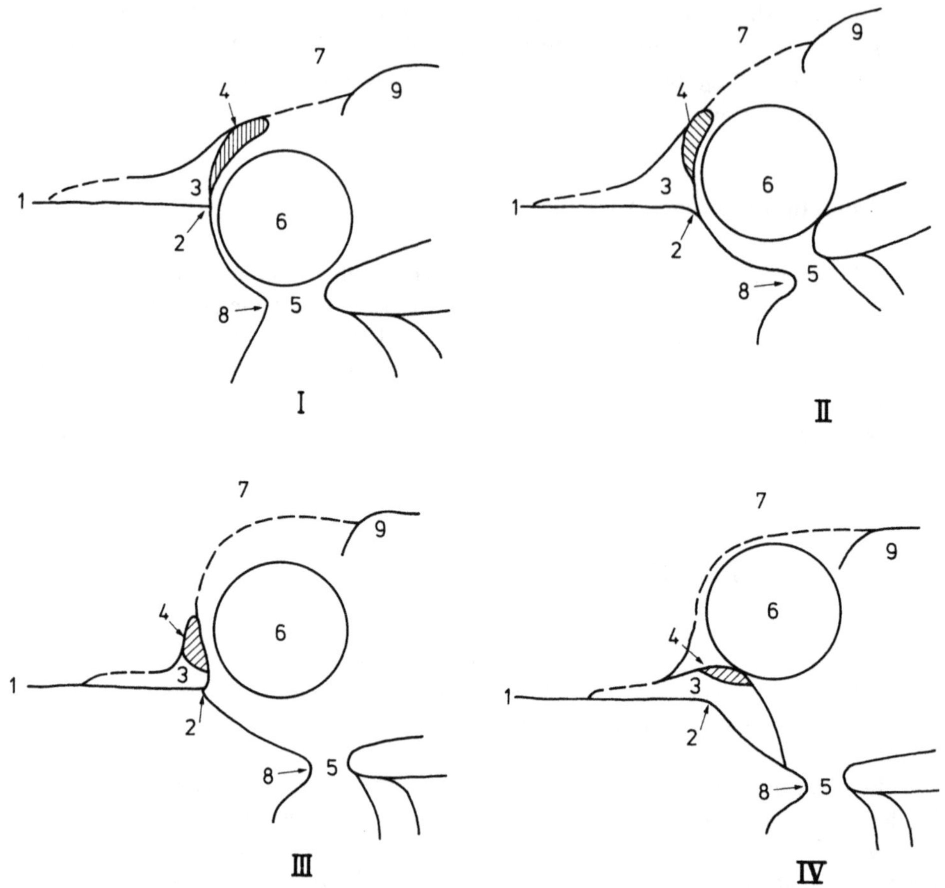

Fig. 1. Graf's original classification of ultrasound findings in the hip of newborns: types I - IV. *1* Iliac wing; *2* bony edge; *3* cartilaginous edge; *4* labrum acetabulare; *5* triad cartilage; *6* cartilaginous femoral head; *7* joint capsule; *8* deepest point of ilium; *9* region of greater trochanter

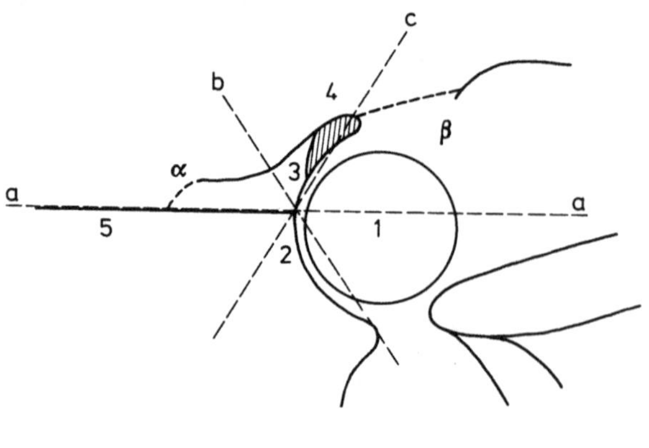

Fig. 2. Diagram of a normal hip joint with angles α and β. *1* femoral head; *2* bony edge; *3* cartilaginous edge; *4* labrum acetabulare; *5* ilium

- Type Ia/b: normal joint at all ages.
- Type IIa: delayed ossification of the cartilaginous edge up to the age of 3 months.
- Type IIb: delayed ossification of the cartilaginous edge in infants of 3 months and older.
- Type IIc: retarded ossification of the cartilaginous edge and small angle α.
- Type D: early dislocation, lateralization of the femoral head.
- Types IIIa/b, IV: different forms of dislocated hips. In *type IIIa* the cartilaginous edge is compressed; in *type IIIb* the cartilaginous edge is compressed and shows histological transformation so that it becomes echoic in the ultrasound picture; in *type IV* the cartilaginous edge is dislocated downwards behind the femoral head.

For the measurement of angles α and β the following three lines are necessary (Fig. 2):

- Line a: between the bony acetabular edge and the insertion of the joint capsule on the iliac wing
- Line b: between the bony acetabular edge and the deepest point of the ilium
- Line c: between the bony acetabular edge and the center of the labrum acetabulare

Angle α is measured between lines a and b, angle β between lines a and c.

6 Technical Requirements for Ultrasound Investigation of the Hip

6.1 Transducer Frequency

For the examination of hip joints in newborns and infants, ultrasound transducers with a frequency of at least 5 MHz are necessary. If a lower frequency is used, the structures of the hip joint are not sufficiently visualized.

Linear arrays, sector scanners and curved arrays can be used. The advantage of linear and curved arrays is better visualization of the subcutaneous tissues. If a sector scanner is used in newborns, a higher frequency (7 MHz and above) should be used or a slice of Reston or Proxon interposed.

6.2 Technique

The easiest position for ultrasound examination of a newborn or infant is the stable lateral position (Fig. 3). The hip to be examined should be uppermost, the patient immobilized with the ipsilateral leg in slight flexion. The scanner is positioned on the greater trochanter if a linear array is used, slightly higher if a sector scanner is used.

The position of the transducer is correct if the ilium is visible as a straight line on the monitor. If the ilium is curved backwards, the scanner is positioned too far dorsally, if curved forwards too far ventrally. The hip joint must be observed in all parts from the ventral to the dorsal acetabular rim.

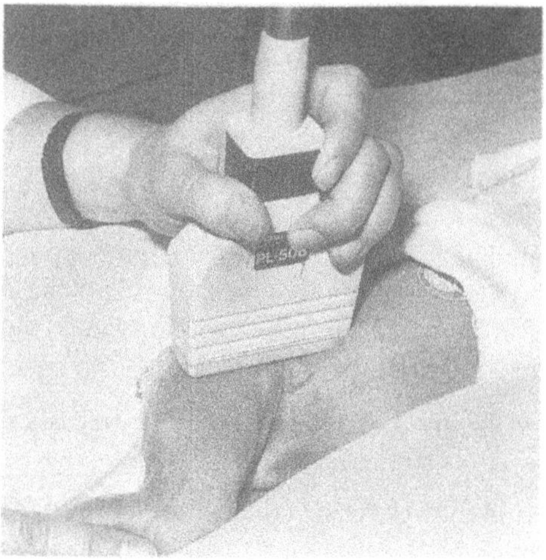

Fig. 3. Patient in stable lateral position, 5-MHz linear array in use

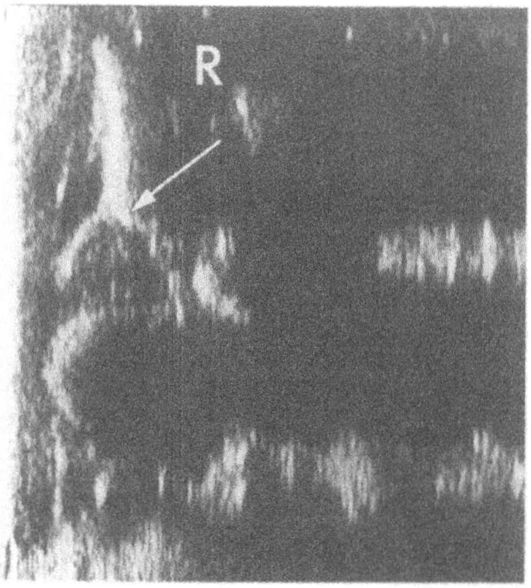

Fig. 4. Right hip of a 4-day-old male newborn, type Ib. Angled/rounded bony edge (*arrow*), central position of femoral head, $\alpha = 68°$, $\beta = 63°$. Picture positioned like a right hip joint on a pelvic roentgenogram

6.3 Documentation

The documentation of ultrasound examinations of the hip has not been uniform. Graf's images are in an upright position showing each hip joint like a right hip joint on a plain X-ray (Fig. 4).

Our images are, as agreed upon for international convenience, all positioned so that the cranial structures are on the left side of the picture. The examined hip must therefore be marked "right" or "left". Each hip joint should be documented at least twice, once with and once without angle measurement.

7 Comparative Postmortem Intraindividual Studies of Hip Joints

In order to establish whether ultrasound of the hip is a reliable diagnostic procedure, we performed comparative intraindividual postmortem studies.

7.1 Patients and Methods

Twenty preterm babies, newborns and young infants were investigated by (a) ultrasound of the hip joints, (b) plain X-ray surveys of the pelvis, (c) ultrasound of the hips after injection of an ultrasound contrast medium (Echovist; experimental trial) and (d) arthrography after intra-articular injection of an iodine-containing conventional contrast medium. Particular attention was paid to the comparison of ultrasound after contrast medium injection and conventional arthrography. The contrast medium was injected in order to visualize the joint cavity, which is not otherwise directly visible on ultrasound. In total, 40 hip joints of preterm babies, newborns, and infants were investigated intra-individually postmortem. The weights and ages of the children are shown in Table 2. The postmortem investigations were carried out between 1 h and 12 h after death.

The heterogeneity of the group enabled evaluation of the typical sonographic and arthrographic findings in preterm babies, newborns and infants.

Table 2. Birthweight and age at the time of investigation

Examined group	Weight (g) at investigation	Age at investigation
Prematures < 30th week of gestation	810 - 1240	hours - 14 days
Prematures 30th - 36th week of gestation	1270 - 2350	hours - 2 days
Newborns	2410 - 3350	hours - 7 days
Infants	3720 - 4910	1 - 3 ½ months

7.2 Results

We investigated 12 preterm babies, four newborns, and four infants between 1 and 3 ½ months of age. The birthweight of the preterm babies and newborns varied between 810 g and 3350 g, the length at birth between 34 cm and 54 cm. Fourteen boys and six girls were examined.

7.2.1 Ultrasound

The ultrasound examination revealed physiologically developed hips, type I or IIa, in 39 of 40 investigations. One right hip showed a complete dislocation, type IV.

Table 3. Distribution of ultrasound hip types on postmortem examination ($n = 40$ hips)

Ultrasound type	Premature <30th week of gestation ($n = 18$)	Premature 30th - 36th week of gestation ($n = 6$)	Newborns ($n = 8$)	Infants ($n = 8$)
Ia	2 (5%)	2 (5%)	3 (7.5%)	5 (12.5%)
Ib	10 (25%)	2 (5%)	1 (2.5%)	1 (2.5%)
IIa	6 (15%)	2 (5%)	3 (7.5%)	2 (5%)
IV	-	-	1 (2.5%)	-
Average diameter (mm)	11	12	14	16

Table 3 demonstrates that especially in preterm babies type IIa hips were often observed; in newborns and infants type I hips were seen in a higher percentage. The newborn with the congenital hip dislocation showed an empty acetabulum which was no longer round, but oval in shape.

The labrum acetabulare could be demonstrated in all type I and IIa hips; in premature babies, however, it was a very tiny structure. The bony acetabulum was regularly formed in all type I and IIa hips. In the one complete dislocation, the bony edge was invisible; the lower ilium could not be seen because of the high position of the femur.

7.2.2 Conventional X-Ray

All roentgenograms of the pelvis were obtained under fluoroscopy. Especially in small preterm babies, the information yielded by conventional plain X-ray surveys was inferior to that rendered by ultrasound of the hip, owing to the latter's better visualization of the cartilage and the soft tissues. The complete dislocation, however, was visible on routine pelvic roentgenograms.

7.2.3 Ultrasound After Intra-articular Injection of Ultrasound Contrast Medium (Ultrasound Arthrography)

After ultrasound examination and pelvic roentgenography 0.2 - 0.5 ml sonographic contrast medium (Echovist) was injected into the hip joints. During the dynamic investigation the distribution of the contrast agent within the joint cavity could be observed. The ultrasound contrast medium marked the capillary joint cavity by small air bubbles; the cartilaginous femoral head was surrounded by these bubbles. The width of the joint cavity was 1 mm in newborns and infants and less than 1 mm in small preterm babies. On the sonographic image the air bubbles can be seen as echoic structures surrounding the cartilaginous femoral head (Fig. 5).

7.2.4 Conventional Arthrography

Arthrography is a well-established method for the diagnosis of congenital hip dislocation. Some orthopaedic surgeons demand diagnostic arthrography before therapy

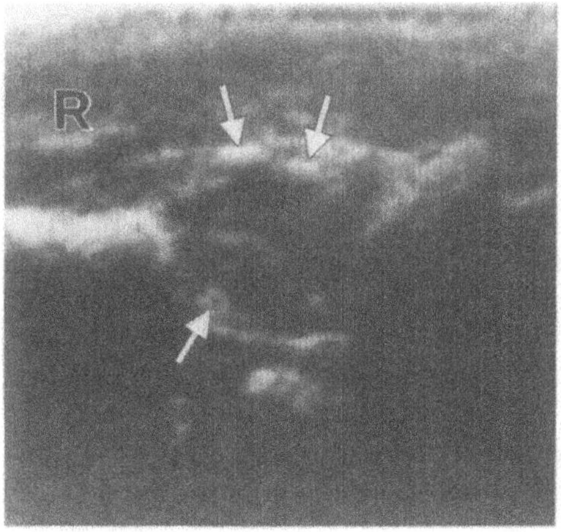

Fig. 5. A right hip joint after intra-articular injection of ultrasound contrast medium: air bubbles surrounding the femoral head (*arrows*)

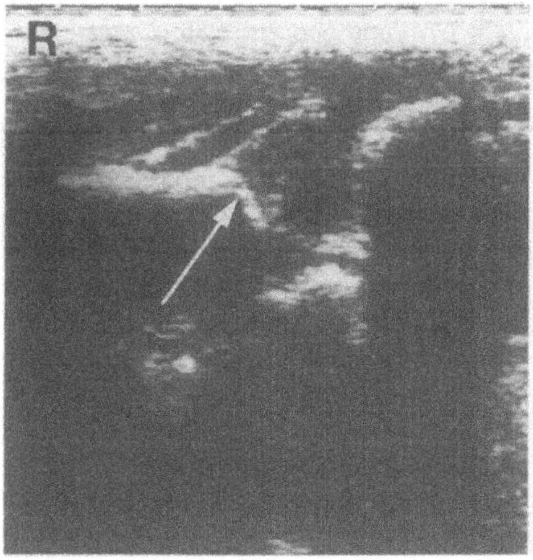

Fig. 6. Right hip of a 6-day-old female newborn. Rounded bony edge (*arrow*), centered femoral head, $\alpha = 56°$, $\beta = 58°$

(*Schwetlick* and *Kasparek* 1969; *Tönnis* 1980). In 39 cases out of 40, the postmortem investigation showed normal findings which correlated with ultrasound types I and IIa. The newborn with the dislocation of the right hip displayed an oval-shaped cartilaginous femoral head and a straightened joint capsule.

Arthrography in preterm babies was technically difficult because of the small joint cavity.

Because of the different imaging techniques the data of X-ray arthrography and ultrasound arthrography are not directly comparable. On the conventional arthrogram all recesses are visible, but partially superimposed, while on the ultrasound scan only one slice of the joint is visible depending on the position of the probe, and owing to the worse spatial resolution the recesses of the joint capsule are not visible. Comparable pictures cannot be obtained by ultrasound ~ and conventional arthrography.

7.3 Discussion

The comparative analysis is based on postmortem investigations of 40 hip joints of preterm babies, newborns and infants. In all cases ultrasound, pelvic roentgenography arthrography after injection of an ultrasonographic contrast medium and conventional arthrography were performed.

In preterm babies born before 30 weeks of gestation the hip joints were generally not fully developed, showing extensive cartilaginous areas. This sonographic finding could not be duplicated using any other diagnostic procedure. On X-ray arthrography, however, a broad labrum acetabulare could be visualized. The position of the femoral head was central in all premature babies.

Comparison of the different diagnostic procedures demonstrates that ultrasound and arthrography are the best for the visualization of an incompletely developed hip joint with persistent extensive areas of cartilage.

In newborns all hip joint structures could be visualized sonographically without the need for intra-articular injection of contrast medium. Pelvic roentgenograms are of no value for the diagnosis of congenital hip dysplasia in preterm babies or newborns (*Ball* and *Kommenda* 1968; *Graf* 1980, 1983a, b, 1985; *Graf* and *Schuler* 1986; *Langer* 1987; *Lefaure* et al. 1985; *Reither* and *Schumacher*; *Schulz* et al. 1986; *Weitzel* et al. 1985). Complete or incomplete unilateral dislocations, however, are visible on plain X-ray surveys.

Our comparative intraindividual study of different diagnostic methods proves that ultrasound is of value for the visualization of the cartilaginous and osseous parts of the neonatal hip joint. Arthrography is also valuable, but invasive, and thus only indicated to answer special questions. Sonographic arthrography, an experimental technique performed in this study to visualize the hip joint cacity directly, probably has no clinical relevance.

8 Comparison of Linear Arrays and Sector Scanners in Ultrasound of the Hip

Comparative studies were done in order to establish which kind of transducer is best for the investigation of hip joints.

8.1 Patients and Methods

The following ultrasound machines were compared:

- Sonoline SL (Siemens) with a 5-MHz linear array and a 5-MHz sector scanner
- SAL 20 A (Toshiba) with a 5-MHz linear array
- Sonodiagnost R 1500 (Philips) with a 5-MHz sector scanner
- Combison 320 (Kraetz) with a 5-MHz sector scanner incorporating an integrated Reston slice

All ultrasound pictures could be magnified by a factor of at least 2.

In an intraindividual comparative study, 50 patients (100 hips) were examined with the 5-MHz sector scanner and the 5-MHz linear array of the Sonoline SL, the 5-MHz linear array of the SAL 20 A and the 5-MHz sector scanner of the Sonodiagnost R 1500.

Thirty other patients (60 hips) were studied with the 5-MHz sector scanner of the Combison 320 and the 5-MHz linear array of the SAL 20 A. The comparison between the image quality of the different ultrasound machines was done subjectively by the examiner.

8.2 Results

The following advantages and disadvantages were observed for 5-MHz linear arrays:

1. The subcutaneous structures are well visible: this is important in the investigation of the hips of newborns and small infants.
2. The examination is easier to perform for inexperienced clinicians.
3. A long (ca. 10 cm) linear array is difficult to use in small newborns and preterm babies.

The analysis of the investigations with the sector scanners showed the following:

1. The application of sector scanners is easier because the scanners are smaller.
2. The subcutaneous structures are not visualized as well as with linear arrays. This is of great importance for low-weight preterm babies.

There was no significant difference in the quality of the linear arrays and sector scanners compared.

8.3 Conclusion

Linear as well as sector tranducers can be used for ultrasound investigation of the hip joint.

9 Comparison of Pelvic Roentgenography and Ultrasound of the Hip Joint

The value of pelvic roentgenography in children up to 3 months of age is low (*Ball* and *Kommenda* 1968; *Graf* 1985; *Imhäuser* 1982; *Palmen* 1984; *Schuster* 1978; *Tönnis* 1976, 1980; *Visser* 1984; *Weitzel* et al. 1985). Before ultrasound of the hip became an established method, high-risk patients were mostly investigated at 3 months of age or older.

9.1 Patients and Methods

In order to compare the value of pelvic roentgenography and ultrasound, 200 infants of 3 - 10 months of age (98 boys and 102 girls) were examined by both methods. All patients

Table 4a. Classification of the acetabular angle. Modified from *Tönnis* and *Brunken* (1968)

Age	Normal findings	
	Males	Females
3 - 6 months	Right: 25 ± 4.7 (max. 29)	21 ± 4.6 (max. 25)
	Left: 26 ± 5.1 (max. 31)	23 ± 4.7 (max. 28)
6 - 12 months	Right: 21 ± 4 (max. 25)	20 ± 4 (max. 24)
	Left: 23 ± 4.1 (max. 27)	23 ± 4.7 (max. 25)

Table 4b. Acetabular angle in the investigated group ($n = 400$)

Age		Normal findings (°)		Pathological findings (°)	
		Female	Male	Female	Male
3 - 6 months	Right:	24 ± 4	22 ± 3	36 ± 4.2	33 ± 2.5
	Left:	25 ± 5.4	22 ± 4.1	38 ± 6	34 ± 4.5
6 - 10 months	Right:	19 ± 3.2	18 ± 5.3	31 ± 4	33 ± 5.8
	Left:	20 ± 5.9	18 ± 4.2	33 ± 2.4	32 ± 3.4

referred for plain X-ray surveys of the pelvis were additionally investigated by ultrasound of the hips. The radiation exposure ruled out a prospective study in an unselected group of patients. The comparative study was done at the time when ultrasound of the hip was introduced as a clinical routine examination.

The plain X-ray studies were analysed with regard to a high or lateral position of the femur. The acetabular angle was measured in all pelvic roentgenograms and classified according to the published data of *Tönnis* and *Brunken* (1968). The normal ranges and our own measurements are listed in Tables 4a and 4b.

The ultrasound findings were classified according to *Graf* (1985). The pelvic roentgenograms were coded numerically: 1, normal findings; 2, suspect findings; 3, pathologic findings. The correlation coefficient between the radiographic and sonographic findings was then calculated:

$$r = \frac{m\,\sigma_x}{\sigma_y}.$$

9.2 Results

Normal findings were observed in 87 % and pathological findings in 13 % of investigated hips. The correlation between ultrasound and plain X-rays as regards correct diagnosis was good ($r = 0.91$; $y = 0.06$, $\delta = 0.97$).

This result proves that all suspect or pathologic radiographic findings can be visualized by ultrasound. It does not, however, demonstrate that ultrasound can visualize soft tissues and cartilage in addition to bony structures.

9.3 Discussion

This intraindividual comparative study shows good agreement between radiographic and sonographic findings in a clinically preselected group of patients. This is demonstrated by a correlation coefficient of $r = 0.91$, meaning that all radiographical abnormalities can be visualized by ultrasound.

Similar results were published by *Schulz* et al. (1986) in his comparative study of plain X-ray surveys and ultrasound of the hip. Thus suspected hip dysplasia or dislocation in infants should be investigated by ultrasound and no longer by pelvic roentgenography.

Another advantage of ultrasound of the hip is the possibility of investigating preterm babies, newborns and infants below 3 months of age, permitting early initiation of therapy in the case of pathology (*Bayer* 1958; *Becker* 1963; *Frischknecht* 1957; *Graf* 1985; *Graf* and *Schuler* 1986; *Haike* 1965; *Palmen* 1984; *Tönnis* 1980).

In view of these results, ultrasound of the hip has been adopted as a routine method in our department, pelvic roentgenography now being employed in only about 5% of cases, namely in children with special clinical problems, such as skeletal dysplasias, and in children, in whom adequate ultrasound investigation is no longer possible (mostly infants of 10 months and older).

10 Ultrasound Screening Programme

10.1 Patients and Methods

In cooperation with the Department of Obstetrics, all newborns were examined randomly by ultrasound of the hip and clinically at the U2 stage (between the 3rd and 10th days of life) from February 1985 to March 1986. The results were compared retrospectively.

A Sonoline SL (Siemens) ultrasound machine with a 5-MHz linear array was used. All newborns were investigated in a stable lateral decubitus position by coronal sections as described by *Graf* (1980; 1983a). In addition, transverse scans of the joints were obtained by a lateral approach.

10.2 Results

A total of 2920 ultrasound examinations were performed in 1460 newborns (718 boys and 742 girls). Most of the children (72.4%) were born in the 39th – 41st week of gestation (Table 5). A familial disposition to congenital dislocation of the hip was established in 61 cases in siblings and in 35 cases in one of the parents. Records of gestation and delivery

Table 5. Gestational age at birth of the babies in the screening programme ($n = 1460$)

Week of gestation	No. of babies	%	Week of gestation	No. of babies	%
31	1	0.1	38	150	10.3
32	3	0.2	39	225	15.4
33	4	0.3	40	459	31.4
34	7	0.5	41	374	25.6
35	7	0.5	42	142	9.7
36	18	1.2	43	15	1.0
37	55	3.8			

Table 6. Distribution of the ultrasound hip types in the postpartum screening programme ($n = 1460$ patients, 2920 hips)

Type	Sex	*n* Hips	%	Type	Sex	*n* Hips	%
Ia	M	480	16.44	IIIa	M	3	0.10
	F	456	15.62		F	8	0.27
Ib	M	640	21.92	IIIb	M	–	–
	F	638	21.85		F	6	0.21
IIa	M	310	10.62	IV	M	–	–
	F	371	12.70		F	2	0.07
IIc	M	–	–	Uncertain	M	3	0.10
	F	3	0.10		F	–	–
D	M	–	–				
	F	–	–				

revealed a normal fetal position in 91.5 %, a breech presentation in 5.7 %, a transverse lie in 0.4 %, and other positions in 2.3 % of cases. Clinical examination at the U2 stage revealed the following:

- Positive Ortolani's sign in seven cases
- Limited abduction of the hip in 34 cases
- Asymmetrical folds in 19 cases

The distribution of ultrasound types of the hip according to Graf is shown in Table 6. Types Ia and Ib (2214 hips) were present in approximately the same proportion of boys and girls, but type IIa (681 hips, Fig. 6) was more frequent in girls. Types IIc (three hips, Fig. 7), IIIa/b (17 hips, Fig. 8) and IV (two hips, Fig. 9) were found only rarely, again mostly in girls.

Patients with type I hips were not reinvestigated, with the exception of those with a familial disposition. To date 277 patients have been reinvestigated by ultrasound, including 190 with type IIa hips (Table 7). One newborn with a type IIc hip was not returned for repeat ultrasound; the parents had refused orthopaedic therapy. All neonates with hips type IIc, IIIa/b and IV were referred to our Department of Orthopaedic Surgery for therapy, which usually took 4 – 12 weeks when started at an early stage.

Table 7. Ultrasound findings in the reinvestigated babies at the first and second control ultrasound examination ($n = 277$)

Findings	Patients	
	n	%
Normal / normalized at first control	229	82.7
Normalized at the second control	42	15.2
Worsened at the first control: → therapy	5	1.8
Uncertainty at control examinations (giant haemangioma)	1	0.4

Table 8. Ultrasound hip types in preterm babies ($n = 230$ hips) and newborns ($n = 2920$ hips)

Type	Preterm babies (%)	Newborns (%)
Ia	14.3	75.8
Ib	33.9	
IIa	51.4	23.3
IIc	0.4	0.1
D	-	-
IIIa/b	-	0.6
IV	-	0.1
Uncertain	-	0.1

All babies undergoing therapy were investigated by ultrasonography weekly until the position of the femoral head had become central relative to the acetabulum.

An additional investigation of 115 preterm babies born between the 28th and 35th week of gestation with birthweights below 2000 g showed type IIa hips in 51% (Table 8). All premature babies had normal clinical findings at the U2 stage. All these type IIa hips developed to become type I joints by 3 – 6 months. This small series demonstrates the significantly higher incidence of type IIa hips in preterm babies than in babies born at term.

10.3 Discussion

Hip sonography has been performed intensively since 1983 by many paediatric radiologists. *Graf's* experience with ultrasonic studies of the hip now exceeds 30 000 examinations (*Graf* 1985; *Graf* and *Schuler* 1986). We have examined more than 12 000 hips of newborns and infants.

The necessity of early treatment in congenital hip dysplasia and dislocation is generally accepted by orthopaedic surgeons (*Becker* 1963; *Graf* 1980, 1983 a, b, 1985; *Graf*

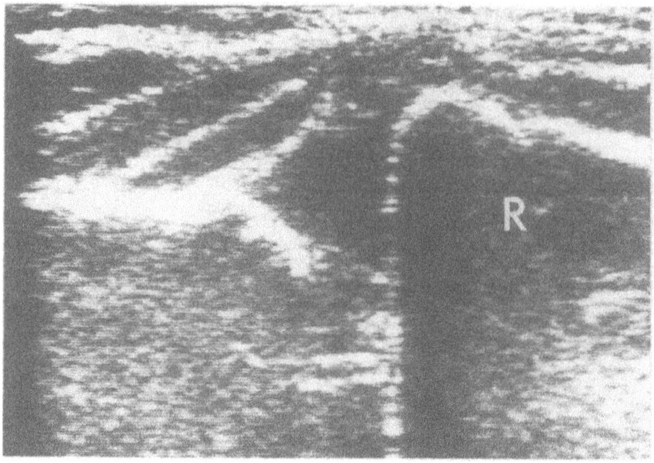

Fig. 7. Right hip of a 2-day-old female newborn, type IIc. Flat bony edge, $\alpha < 50°$, $\beta > 55°$

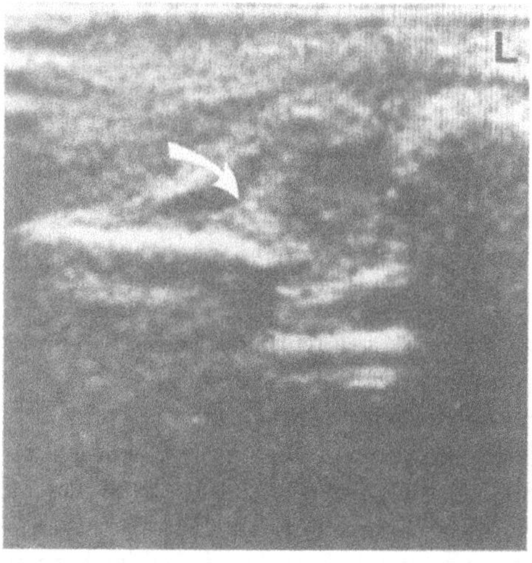

Fig. 8

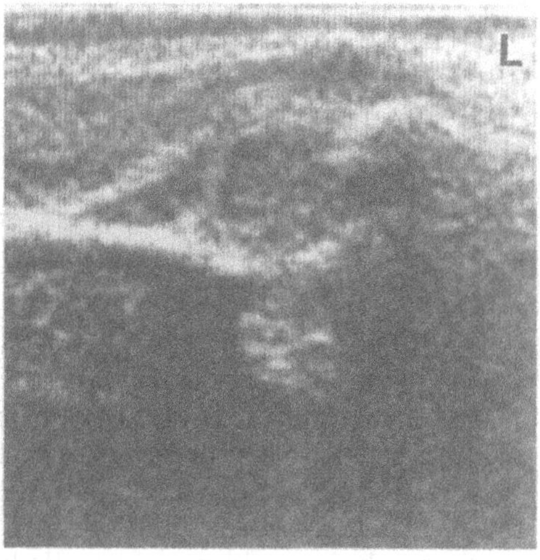

Fig. 9

Fig. 8. Left hip of a 2-day-old female neonate, type IIIb. Flat bony edge, compressed and echoic cartilaginous edge (*arrow*), dislocated femoral head

Fig. 9. Left hip of a 1-day-old female newborn, type IV. Bony edge invisible, cartilaginous edge displaced into the acetabulum, complete dislocation of the femoral head

and *Schuler* 1986; *Haike* 1965; *Schuler* and *Rossak* 1984; *Tönnis* 1980). Studies in Sweden and the Netherlands (*Palmen* 1984; *Rosen* 1962; *Visser* 1984) have demonstrated the importance of accurate and meticulous clinical examination. The significance of the examiner's personal experience has been emphasized by *Palmen* (1984) and *Visser* (1984).

As a rule, complete dislocation of the hip can be readily diagnosed clinically. In contrast, however, early types of hip dysplasia may escape diagnosis by clinical methods. For many years the only imaging procedure was roentgenography of the pelvis, in the form of plain film studies or hip joint arthrography. In Germany, general X-ray screening of all infants aged 3 - 4 months had been banned in 1970 by the German Radiological Society (DRG) because of the exposure to radiation (*Frik* 1972). In contrast to this, French authors reported the results of radiographic screening in infants up to 3 months of age in 1985 (*Lefaure* et al. 1985). The authors discussed X-ray screening of the hip in spite of the accumulated experience with sonography.

In Sweden, the Netherlands and the United Kingdom hip sonography is only now being introduced. In the United States, reports of initial studies of ultrasound of the hip in small groups of patients have appeared (*Boal* and *Schwenkter* 1985; *Morin* et al. 1985; *Novick* et al. 1983).

In 1985 a committee of experts recommended on behalf of the WHO and the European Community that all newborns should be examined clinically. General screening of newborns by X-ray or ultrasound was not agreed (H. *Fendel*, personal communication, April 1986).

In our study we found that 32 % of hips were type Ia and 44 % type Ib, a physiological variant. It has now become clear that a control ultrasound examination is not required in type Ib hips (*Graf* and *Schuler* 1986; *Langer* 1987; *Schulz* et al. 1986). On the basis of our results we consider that type I hips should only be reviewed in cases of familial disposition or of breech or transverse presentation at birth. In our screening programme type IIa hips were found in 23 % of cases. This type is also physiological in newborns and should develop to become type I within 3 months. Type IIa should be reinvestigated by ultrasound, however, because a hip dislocation may develop without recognizable clinical findings (*Graf* 1985; *Hellige* 1986; *Reither* and *Schumacher* 1985; *Weitzel* et al. 1985). The incidence of type IIa in our patients (23 %) is about the same as in Graf's screening programme. In contrast, *Hellige* (1986) observed type IIa hips in only 2 % of cases. In his screening programme, however, only 200 of the hips examined (about 10 %) were measured. He surveyed type IIa hips until they had developed to become type I. *Schulz* et al. (1986), on the other hand, maintain that type IIa hips need not be reinvestigated.

In our patients, 98 % of type IIa hips developed to type I. The remaining 2 % showed constant or worsened findings, and orthopaedic therapy was initiated. Our ultrasound study in preterm babies shows that in this group the development of the hip joint is physiologically delayed.

A comparison of the clinical and sonographic data confirmed the high diagnostic value of Ortolani's sign in the hands of experienced paediatricians. Five patients with positive Ortolani's sign showed hip joint pathology in our group of newborns. No diagnostic significance, however, is attributed to asymmetrical folds or to limited abduction in the neonatal period. Only two of our patients showed abnormal ultrasonographic findings without clinical signs and without a predisposing intrauterine position. These cases can now be indentified by ultrasound.

11 Conclusions

1. Ultrasound of the hip joint is a valuable diagnostic procedure in the hands of experienced physicians.
2. Ultrasound of the hip should be performed in high-risk babies shortly after birth.
3. The following features place patients in the high-risk group:

– positive Ortolani's or Barlow's sign
– familial disposition
– predisposing intrauterine position
– twins
– meningomyelocele or other neurological diseases or malformations
– shortening of one leg
– foot abnormalities
(– limited abduction, asymmetrical folds)

4. Ultrasound of the hip is suitable as a screening procedure only if sufficient expertise and adequate ultrasound apparatus are available.

References

Ball F, Kommenda K (1968) Sources of error in the roentgen evaluation of the hip in infancy. Ann Radiol (Paris) 11: 298-303
Barlow TG (1962) Early diagnosis and treatment of congenital dislocation of the hip. J Bone Joint Surg (Br) 44: 292-301
Bayer R (1958) Über den Wert obligater Röntgenuntersuchungen bei Säuglingen zur Früherfassung der kongenitalen Hüftgelenksluxation. Wien Med Wochenschr 108: 186
Becker F (1963) Prophylaxe und Frühbehandlung der kongenitalen Dysplasie des Hüftgelenks. Arch Orthop Unfall-Chir 55: 218-229
Boal DKB, Schwenkter EP (1985) The infant hip: assessment with real-time US. Radiology 157: 667-672
Dörr WM (1966) Zur Frühest- und Frühdiagnose der sogenannten angeborenen Hüftgelenksluxation. Dtsch Med Wochenschr 91: 168-173
Dunn PM (1969) Congenital dislocation of the hip (CDH): necropsy studies at birth. Proc Soc Med 62: 1035-1037
Dunn PM (1974) Congenital postural deformities: further perinatal associations. Proc Soc Med 67: 1174-1178
Faber A (1938) Untersuchungen über die Ätiologie und Pathogenese der angeborenen Hüftverrenkung. Thieme, Leipzig
Frik W (1972) Reihenuntersuchungen der Hüftgelenke bei Säuglingen und Strahlenschutz. Fortschr Röntgenstr 116: 453-455
Frischknecht W (1957) Zur Frühdiagnose und Pathogenese der kongenitalen Hüftluxation. Schweiz Med Wochenschr 3: 64-66
Gladel W (1983) Luxationshüfte und Vorsorgeuntersuchung. Z Orthop 121: 613-618
Graf R (1980) The diagnosis of congenital hip-joint dislocation by the ultrasonic combound treatment. Arch Orthop Traumat Surg 97: 117-133
Graf R (1983a) Grundprinzipien der sonographischen Hüftgelenksdysplasie bei Säuglingen. Orthop Praxis 12: 933-941
Graf R (1983b) New possibilities for the diagnosis of congenital hip joint dislocation by ultrasonography. J Pediatr Orthop 3: 354-359
Graf R (1985) Sonographie der Säuglingshüfte. Enke, Stuttgart

Graf R, Schuler P (1986) Die Säuglingshüfte im Ultraschallbild: ein Atlas. Edition Medizin, Weinheim
Haike HJ (1965) Früherkennung und Frühbehandlung der sogenannten kongenitalen Hüftluxation und Hüftdysplasie. Dtsch Med Wochenschr 50: 1253 - 1257
Hellige R (1986) Erfahrungen mit der Ultraschalluntersuchung der Säuglingshüfte in der ersten Lebenswoche bei 1000 Säuglingen. In Otto RC, Schnaars P (Hrsg) Ultraschall-Diagnostik 85. Thieme, Stuttgart
Imhäuser G (1982) Irrtümer in der Beurteilung kindlicher Hüftgelenke durch die konventionelle Röntgentechnik. Z Orthop 120: 93 - 99
Izadpanah M (1979) Die Bedeutung der Kombination von Arthrographie und Spezialaufnahme bei der Luxationshüfte. Z Orthop 117: 816 - 820
Langer R (1987) Ultrasonic investigation of the hip in newborns in the diagnosis of congenital hip dislocation. Skeletal Radiol 16: 275 - 279
Langer R, Kaufmann HJ (1986) Ultrasound screening of the hip in newborns and comparative post mortem studies of the hip by ultrasound and arthrography. Pediatr Radiol 16: 343
Lefaure C, Maccia C, Corlobe F (1985) An overview of the CDH. Radiological screening in France. Pediatr Radiol 15: 275
Mitchell GP (1972) Problems in the early diagnosis and management of congenital dislocation of the hip. J Bone Joint Surg [Br] 54: 4 - 12
Moore SG, Gooding CA, Brasch RC, Edwards DE (1985) The evaluation of congenital dislocation of the hip by magnetic resonance imaging. Pediatr Radiol 15: 280
Morin C, Harcke HT, MacEwen GD (1985) The infant hip: real-time US assessment of acetabular development. Radiology 157: 673 - 677
Newberg AH, Munn CS, Robbins AH (1985) Complications of arthrography. Radiology 155: 605 - 606
Novick G, Ghelman B, Schneider M (1983) Sonography of the neonatal and infant hip. Am J Roentgenol 141: 639 - 645
Palmen K (1984) Prevention of congenital dislocation of the hip. Acta Orthop Scand 55 [Suppl]: 208
Reither M, Schumacher R (1985) Ultraschalldiagnostik der Hüftgelenksdysplasie. Pädiat Prax 31: 557 - 566
Rosen S (1962) Diagnosis and treatment of congenital dislocation of the hip joint in the newborn. J Bone Joint Surg [Br] 44: 284 - 291
Schuler P, Rossak K (1984) Sonographische Verlaufskontrollen von Hüftreifungsstörungen. Z Orthop 122: 136 - 141
Schulz RD, Zieger M, Haas H (1986) The present standard of ultrasonography in newborn and young infant hips. Pediatr Radiol 16: 343
Schuster W (1978) Radiologic interpretation of dysplasia of the acetabulum. In: Weil UH (ed) Progress in orthopaedic surgery, vol 2 Springer, Berlin Heidelberg, New York, pp 73 - 84
Schwetlick W, Kasparek HG (1969) Die Harmonisierung von Doppelkontrastarthrogrammen kindlicher Hüftgelenke. Z Orthop 106: 527 - 535
Sinios A (1969) Diagnose und Therapie der sogenannten Hüftdysplasie. Pädiat Prax 8: 641 - 654
Strife JL, Towbin R, Crawford A (1984) Hip arthrography in infants and children: the inferomedial approach. Radiology 152: 536
Thomas G (1960) Zur Technik der Arthrographie des Hüftgelenkes bei der Lux. cox. congenitalis. Z Orthop 92: 306 - 308
Tönnis D (1976) Die angeborene Hüftdysplasie läßt sich in den ersten Lebensmonaten nicht statistisch abgrenzen! Arch Orthop Unfall-Chir 85: 237 - 240
Tönnis D (1980) Die heutigen Verfahren zur Frühbehandlung der Hüftdysplasie und der kongenitalen Hüftluxation. Dtsch Ärztebl 12: 747 - 753
Tönnis D, Brunken D (1968) Eine Abgrenzung normaler und pathologischer Hüftpfannendachwinkel zur Diagnose der Hüftdysplasie. Arch Orthop Unfall-Chir 64: 197 - 228
Tredwell SJ, Bell HM (1981) Efficacy of neonatal hip examination. J Pediatr Orthop 1: 61 - 65
Visser JD (1984) Functional treatment of congenital dislocation of the hip. Acta Orthop Scand 55 [Suppl]: 206
Weitzel D, Humburg C, Peters H (1985) Hüftgelenkssonographie. Der Kinderarzt 16: 1191 - 1198
Wynne-Davies R (1970) A family study of neonatal and late-diagnosis congenital dislocation of the hip. J Med Genet 7: 315 - 333

Defecography: A Supplementary Diagnostic Asset in the Study of the Disorders of Defecation

P.H.G. Mahieu [1]

1 Introduction

The proper treatment of functional disorders of rectal evacuation requires that the diagnosis be as accurate as possible. To supplement anamnesis and clinical examination, techniques such as anorectal manometry and electromyography have been developed. Conventional radiology makes its contribution through defecography. This technique allows two types of approach to rectal evacuation, one static and the other dynamic. The static examination essentially produces additional refinements as to the position of the opacified anorectal system against the pelvic bones, both at rest and during straining. The dynamic examination evaluates the movement of the rectal and anal lining, both at rest and during straining, as well as the movement of the muscular pelvic floor – in particular of the puborectal muscle.

As early as 1964, *Burhenne* emphasized the fact that after barium enema the evacuation of the contrast material occurs without the radiologist making use of this moment in the examination, which in fact can provide much very useful diagnostic material (*Burhenne* 1964). Even though some of the first radiologists did study the evacuation of liquid barium (*Brown* 1965; *Burhenne* 1964), there were others who preferred to render the feces opaque by having their patients eat meals with barium sulfate added for 3 consecutive days (*Phillips* and *Edwards* 1965). This rather impractical technique was modified by administering a more dense barium mixture to the patients rectally (*Kerremans* 1969). Radiocinematography was then used as a means of recording (*Broden* and *Snellman* 1968; *Kerremans* 1969). This technique involves the inconvenience of relatively high irra-

[1] Université Catholique de Louvain, Institut Chirurgical de Bruxelles, Radiology Department UCL, Square Marie-Louise 59, 1040-Brussels, Belgium

diation and the need for a sophisticated set of apparatus which is no longer widely available. More recently, two methods of opacification have been developed - one, balloon proctography, at St Mark's Hospital in London (*Preston* et al. 1982) and the other, called defecography, under development since 1978, at the *Institut Chirurgical de Bruxelles* (Surgical Institute of Brussels) (*Mahieu* et al. 1981, 1984a,b; *Mahieu* 1983). Ten years of experience indicate that defecography offers a number of advantages on the level of precision diagnosis, while at the same time it constitutes a technique that can be used in routine situations.

2 Method

Both the static and the dynamic examination are preceded by the opacification of the anorectal system.

Let us recall that in the balloon proctography technique a lubricated radiotransparent balloon is mounted on a catheter with which it communicates. It is then introduced into the rectum and filled with liquid barium. Slight traction on the catheter is sufficient to draw the extreme point of the opaque balloon into the anal canal. The contours of the rectal ampulla and of the anal canal can thus be grossly visualized, both at rest and at the beginning of straining, as long as the balloon has not been expelled.

Defecography (*Mahieu* et al. 1981, 1984a,b; *Mahieu* 1983) consists of opacifying the rectum with a paste composed of a mixture of liquid barium and potato starch. After heating, this mixture forms a paste with the usual semi-solid consistency of the feces. A volume of about 250 ml of this paste is introduced into the rectum by means of an injector. To make the anal canal opaque the paste is continuously injected while the extremity of the injector is progressively drawn out through the anus. For improved coating and for a sharper outline of the rectal mucosa, a concentrated suspension of barium is placed in the anal catheter and injected into the rectum before the paste is injected. In order to improve the quality of the radiographs, a special seat, conceived and utilized since 1978 (*Mahieu* et al. 1981), permits the collection of the contrast material evacuated during the examination. This seat is composed of a set of superposed air chambers, filled only with water and connected with one another by a plexiglass cylinder. The central orifice is equipped with a disposable plastic bag, which is thrown away immediately after the examination. Thus the defecography can take place in hygienic conditions, completely acceptable both for the patient and the medical staff.

The advantage of the presence of water in the air chambers comes from the fact that it has an absorption of X-rays practically identical with that of the structures which are situated in the anal region and could possibly prolapse under the gluteal region. In other words, this technique allows us to produce radiographs which are more uniformly exposed.

The data can be recorded on standard film, video tape, by radiocinematography or by 70- or 100-mm ampliphotography. Usually, we expose a series of 100-mm films at a rate of one or two per second during the peak of the session, with a few standard films to enlarge the field and obtain skeletal reference points (pubis, coccyx).

It is sometimes useful to opacify the vaginal lumen by means of a compress soaked with a contrast medium; this enables better observation of the movements of the rectovaginal septum.

3 Static Examination

Thanks to the technique described it is possible to carry out a static examination from the side with the patient in a sitting position. The static examination aims essentially at determining the position of the anorectal junction in relation to the pubococcygeal line, the anorectal angle at rest and the behavior of the anal sphincter, also at rest.

The *pubococcygeal line* has most often been described as the line connecting the anterior and superior edges of the pubic symphysis to the distal end of the coccyx (*Parks* et al. 1966). The length of a perpendicular line beginning at the pubococcygeal line and descending to the anorectal junction provides a measure of the pelvic floor descent at rest (Fig. 1). Measurement of the same line during straining is also possible (Fig. 2) and the difference between the length of the lines during straining and at rest yields the pelvic floor descent during straining.

The significance of the *anorectal angle* (ARA) is that it seems to be a good measure of the tonic activity of the puborectal muscle. Let us recall that this muscle forms a sling, attaching at the level of the pubic symphysis and supporting the anorectal junction posteriorly. This muscle has the peculiarity of being tonically contracted when at rest, and thus it induces an angulation, the ARA, between the axis of the anal canal and the axis of the rectum, which is taken to be the tangent to the posterior edge of the distal part of the rectal ampulla.

The important role of the puborectal muscle in anal continence, described by *Parks* et al. (1966), is based on the phenomenon of the flap valve: at rest, the muscle is contracted and allows the anterior distal rectal aspect to take up a position opposite to the internal end of the anal canal, rather like a lid. Any increase in abdominal pressure reinforces the efficiency of the lid. When the puborectal muscle relaxes, which normally occurs during

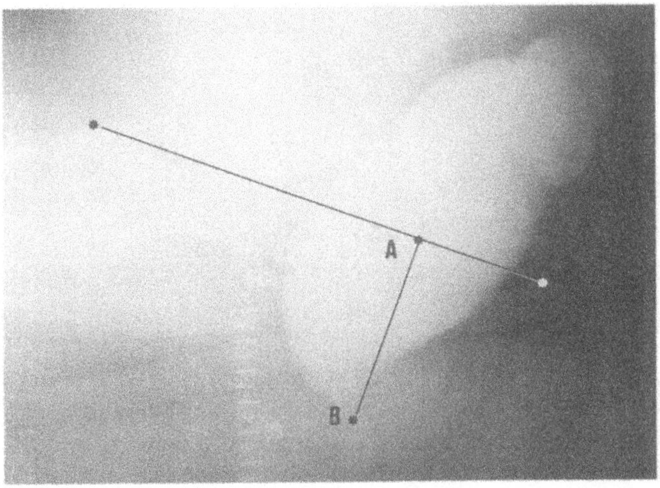

Fig. 1. Normal pelvic floor descent at rest. The descent is represented by the length of the line *AB* joining the pubococcygeal line (*A*) and the anorectal junction (*B*). This distance is not greater than 8.5 cm in a normal patient. The distance can be read from the scale of the radiopaque lath

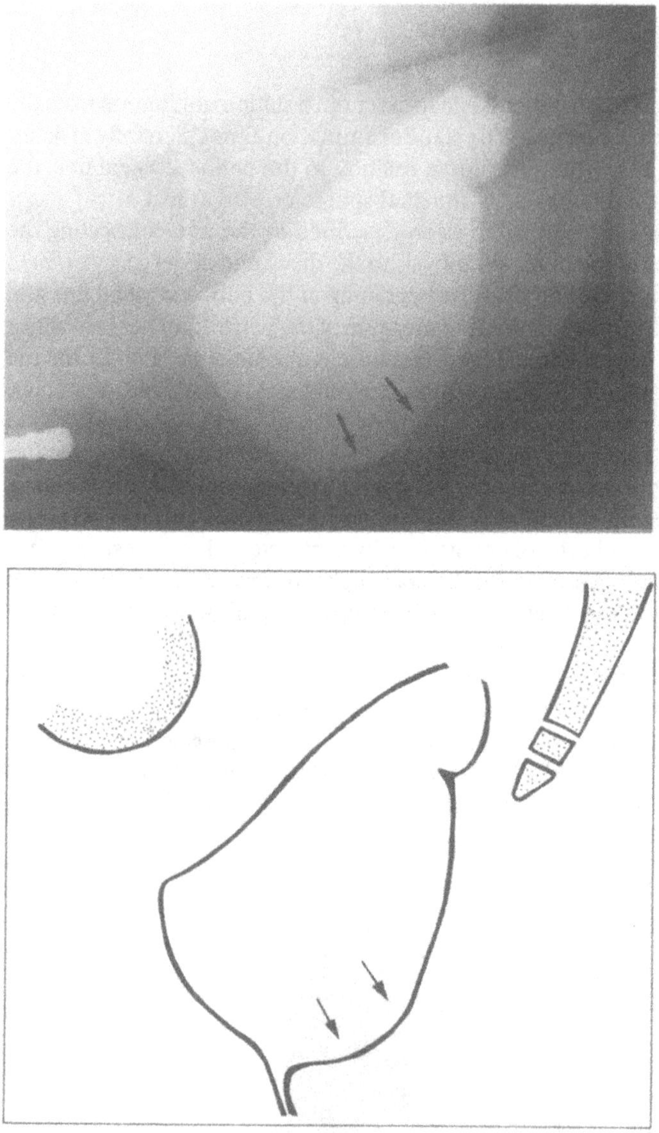

Fig. 2. Abnormal pelvic floor descent during straining, associated with a bulging of the posterior pelvic floor (*arrows*)

voluntary straining, the ARA opens, the valve phenomenon can no longer take place and the emptying of the rectum is made possible by increased abdominal pressure. The valve phenomenon must be considered together with the complementary role of the anal sphincter itself in order to fully explain fecal continence.

The *behavior of the anal sphincter* can be evaluated essentially in terms of its degree of opening, which is an indirect indication of its muscular tonicity.

4 Dynamic Examination

The dynamic study is an essential part of the overall examination because it reveals the anomalies of the anorectal system which arise during and at the end of evacuation. It appraises not only the movements of the rectum and of the anal canal, but also the speed of rectal evacuation, the significance of any possible residue, the value of the ARA during the process of emptying, the degree of resistance offered by the muscular pelvic floor to the pressure produced to obtain rectal evacuation, and the degree of opening of the anal canal. All these data improve the definition of rectal evacuation before considering what treatment is appropriate for the functional disorders.

5 Results

5.1 Static Examination

5.1.1 Pubococcygeal Line and Pelvic Floor Descent

To our knowledge, no study has yet been performed with the aim of precise quantitative assessment of pelvic floor descent, at least not in the sitting position. When *Parks* described the syndrome of the descending perineum (*Parks* et al. 1966), he made the measurements with the patients reclining in a left lateral position. This seems less physiological than the sitting position, as the pelvic floor is not put under pressure. The left lateral reclining position seems equally unsuited for good rectal evacuation.

It seems that, on average, the normal pelvic floor does not descend more than 3 - 3.5 cm during straining compared with its position at rest (*Mahieu* 1987). This value is thus taken as the maximum normal limit for pelvic floor descent during straining. In our experience, the normal value of the pelvic floor descent at rest is 8.5 cm (*Bartram* and *Mahieu* 1985) (Fig. 1).

5.1.2 Anorectal Angle

The value of the ARA at rest has been described as varying from 60° to 105° (*Hardcastle* and *Parks* 1970). Our own studies (*Mahieu* 1983; *Mahieu* et al. 1984a) indicate an ARA of 91.96° ± 1.52° (mean ± SEM) in a group of 56 patients at rest. In the same normal group, the ARA during straining was 136.76° ± 1.51°.

An increase of the ARA at rest is observed in incontinence. In a group of 19 incontinent patients, the ARA was 129.74° ± 2.84° at rest, about 38° more than in the normal patients (*Mahieu* et al. 1984a). However, the existence of an external rectal prolapse or of an intra-anal rectal intussusception is also associated with a significant increase of the ARA at rest (*Mahieu* et al. 1984b).

5.1.3 Behavior of Anal Sphincter

The behavior of the anal sphincter can be roughly appraised on the basis of the width of the column of contrast medium with which it is filled. In the case of chronic anal distension, which often accompanies incontinence, the anal canal, being filled with a relatively broad barium column, is opaque at rest and during straining.

5.2 Dynamic Examination

5.2.1 Normal Defecogram

At the moment of rectal evacuation, the following elements are consistently observed in normal patients and can be taken as the criteria of a normal defecogram: an increase in the ARA, on average, from 92° to 137°; diminution of the imprint left by the puborectal muscle at the level of the posterior side of the anorectal junction; broad opening of the anal canal; complete or practically complete emptying of the rectum; and appropriate resistance by the pelvic floor to the forces exerted to achieve the evacuation of the rectal contents (*Mahieu* et al. 1984a) (Fig. 3).

5.2.2 Principal Radiologically Detectable Disorders of Rectal Evacuation

Intussusception and Prolapse of Rectum. According to some authors (*Broden* and *Snellman* 1968), complete rectal prolapse only constitutes the end-point, the last degree of severity, of the phenomenon of invagination of the rectal wall. In our opinion, different stages can be distinguished (Table 1). *Simple rectal intussusception* corresponds to simple invagination of the rectal wall. This invagination is identified radiologically by the development of a fold which is either lateral, most often anterolateral (*Mahieu* et al. 1984b), or circumferential right from the outset. The fold becomes progressively accentuated and constitutes the starting point for an invagination which remains localized in the rectal lumen. In *rectal intra-anal intussusception* the invagination goes beyond the internal anal margin and extrudes into the anal canal without exteriorizing (Figs. 4A, 6). Finally, *external rectal prolapse* consists of the exteriorization of the invagination through the anal canal. This exteriorization may be spontaneously reversible, the prolapse shrinking as soon as the straining stops, or the manual intervention of the patient may be necessary after the emptying of the rectum.

Rectocele. Radiologically, a rectocele is seen as a progressive depression of the anterior rectal wall and of the rectovaginal septum under the abdominal pressure which pushes

Table 1. Principal defecation disorders radiologically detectable by defecography

Intussusception and prolapse of the rectum
- simple rectal intussusception
- rectal intra-anal intussusception
- external rectal prolapse, manually or spontaneously reversible
Rectocele
Dyskinesia of the puborectal muscle
Descending perineum
Incontinence
Association of several disorders

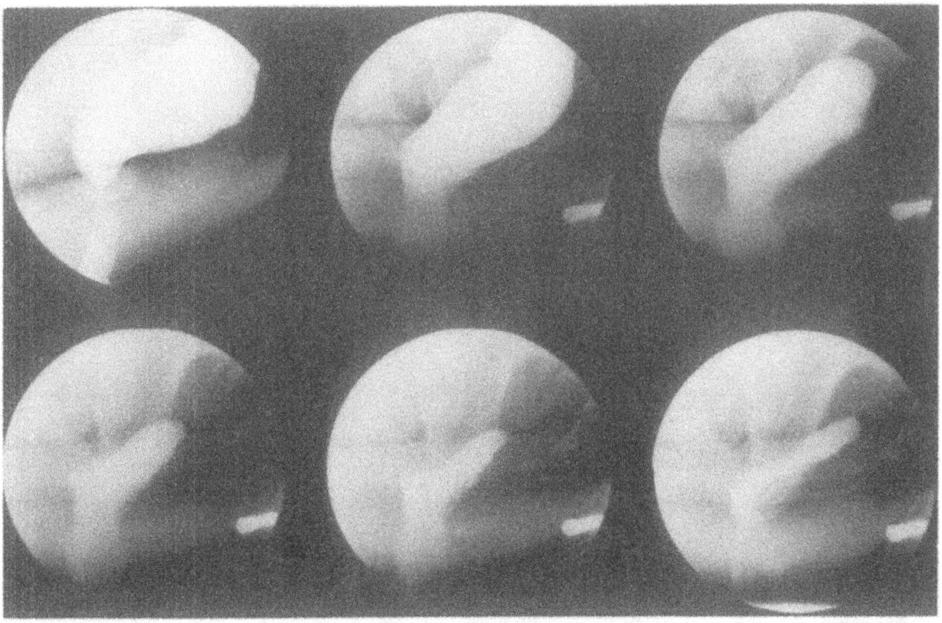

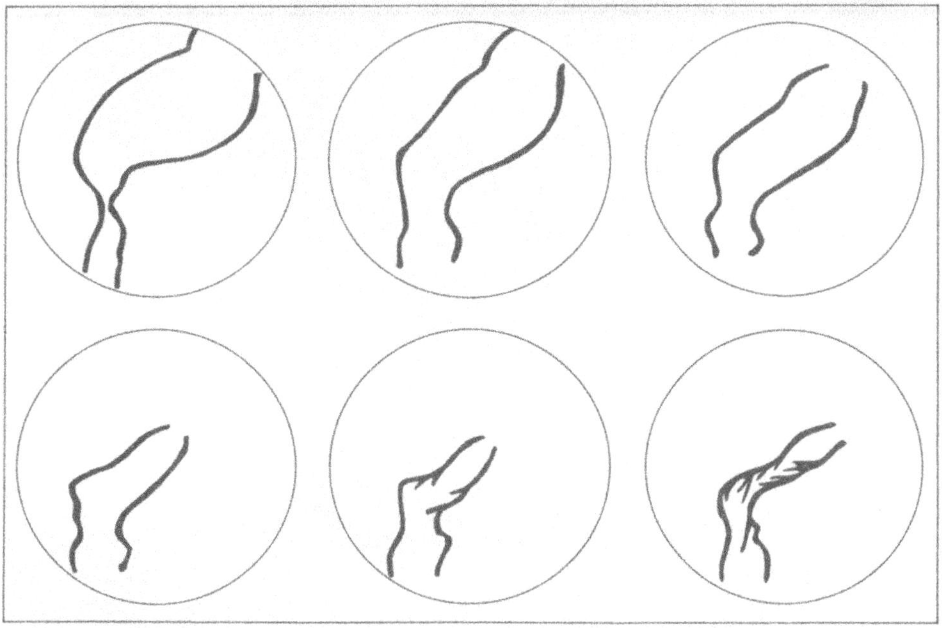

Fig. 3. Normal defecogram (read from left to right and top to bottom). During defecation an increase of the ARA is observed along with a decrease of the imprint of the puborectal muscle on the posterior lining of the anorectal junction, opening of the anal canal, complete evacuation and firm resistance by the pelvic floor

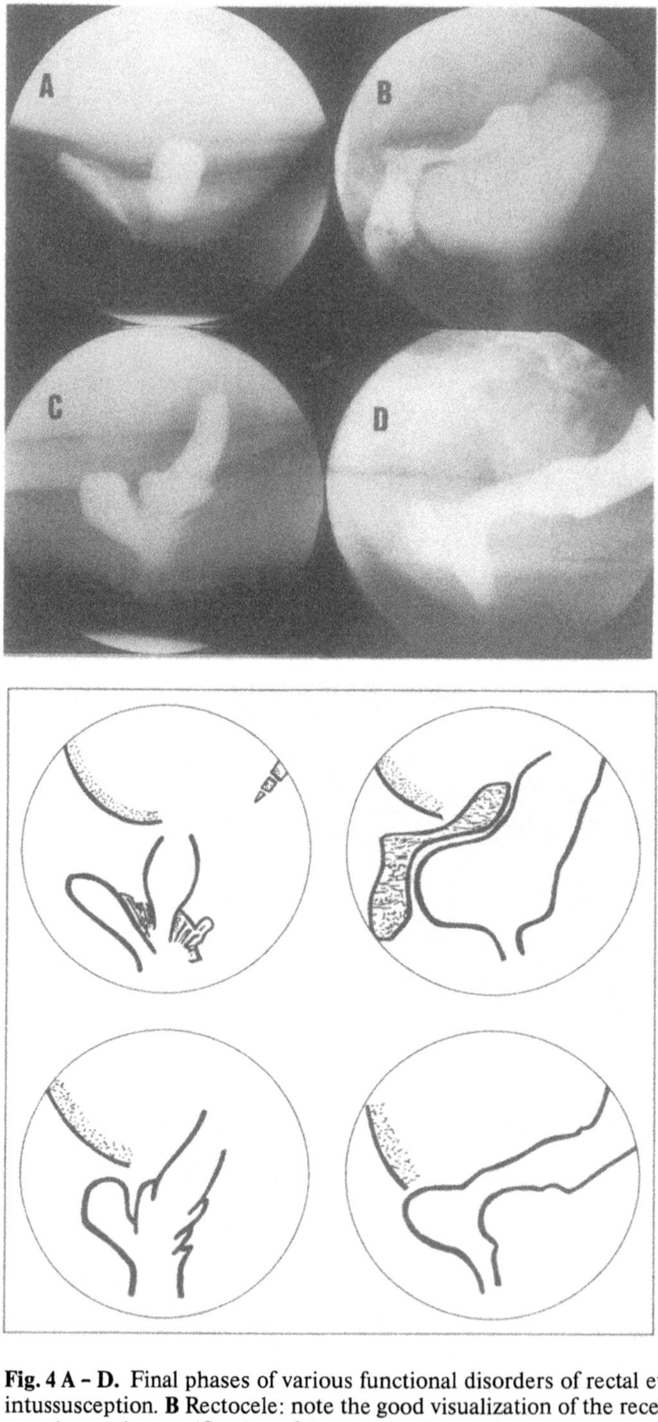

Fig. 4 A – D. Final phases of various functional disorders of rectal evacuation. **A** Intra-anal rectal intussusception. **B** Rectocele: note the good visualization of the recession of the rectovaginal septum due to the opacification of the vagina. **C** Association between a simple rectal intussusception and a small rectocele. **D** Hypertonicity of the puborectal sling: the ARA remains acute, and evacuation is difficult and largely imcomplete

the fecal bolus forward. This depression transforms progressively into a true anterior sacculation in which some of the contrast material which may have persisted, is finally isolated, while the rest of the rectal lumen can be completely evacuated (Fig. 4B). As soon as the straining ceases, the elasticity of the rectal walls makes the opaque sequestrum come back into the rectal lumen (Fig. 5). The persistence of a rectal residue then causes a new urge to evacuate the bowels a relatively short time after the first evacuation.

Association Between Intussusception and Rectocele. A rectocele is often associated with a discrete anterior rectal intussusception. More rarely, it may be associated with a circumferential intussusception. It is, moreover, conceivable that this image sometimes corresponds to a simple mucous prolapse rather than to a true intussusception affecting the entire thickness of the rectal wall (Figs. 4C, 6).

Dyskinesia of the Puborectal Muscle. This dyskinesia most often consists of a hypertonia which can either be intermittent or constant during the entire period of straining. It translates radiologically as an accentuation of the posterior impression at the level of the anorectal junction and as an absence of opening, or even diminution of the ARA during straining. This hypertonicity constitutes an obstacle to normal rectal evacuation which leads to a more intense and prolonged straining, despite the resistance linked to the abnormal contraction of the puborectal muscle (Fig. 4D). Some authors (*Rutter* and *Riddell* 1975) regard this as the probable origin of the solitary rectal ulcer syndrome. In our own study of a group of 43 cases of solitary rectal ulcer, we found only four cases of functional disorders of the puborectal muscle in the form of hypertonicity, while noting 19 cases of external rectal prolapse, five of simple rectal intussusception and 10 of intra-anal rectal intussusception (*Mahieu* 1986).

Descending Perineum. Pelvic floor descent of more than 3 – 3.5 cm from the anorectal junction during straining relative to the position at rest seems to be pathological (*Mahieu* 1987) (Fig. 2). This abnormal descent of the pelvic floor during straining is usually observed in patients presenting the syndrome of the descending perineum (*Parks* et al. 1966).

6 Discussion

We would emphasize the fact that at the beginning of our study – and still now, though to a lesser degree because of the clinician's better knowledge of these functional disorders – defecography detected a number of external prolapses which were not diagnosed as such over several clinical and endoscopic examinations (*Mahieu* et al. 1981). Although the detection of external rectal prolapses has now been improved thanks to more thorough clinical examination, simple or intra-anal rectal intussusception remains a particularly interesting field of application for defecography since its positive demonstration is not otherwise possible. The same holds true for functional disorders of the puborectal sling and of the muscular pelvic floor.

The rival *balloon proctography* technique is neat and simple to carry out, but it must be recognized that defecography offers certain advantages: more precise data as to the movements of the rectal lining and the existence or otherwise of an intussusception or a

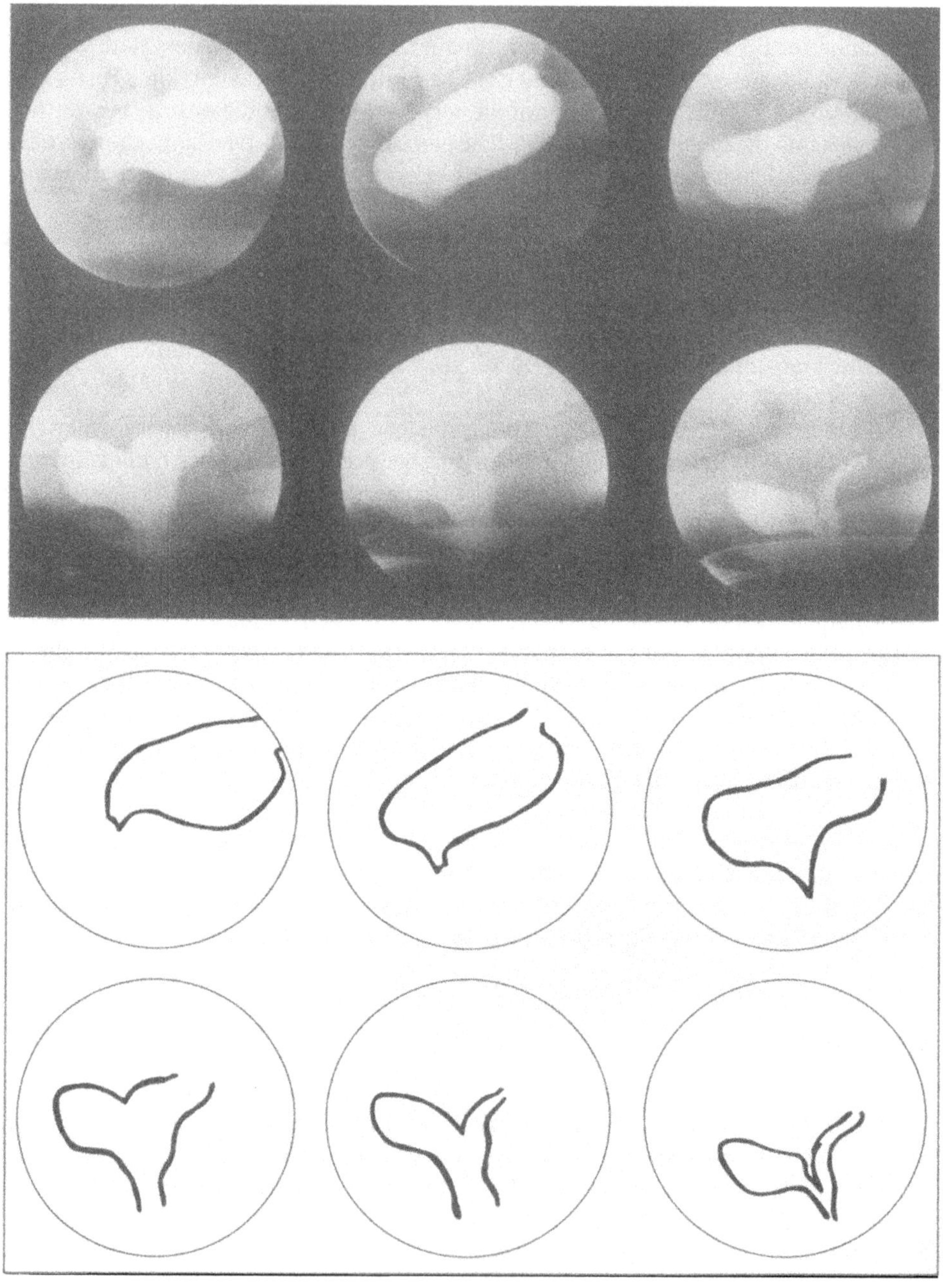

Fig. 5. Rectocele. An anterior rectal sacculation develops progressively and at the end of the evacuation isolates part of the rectal contents

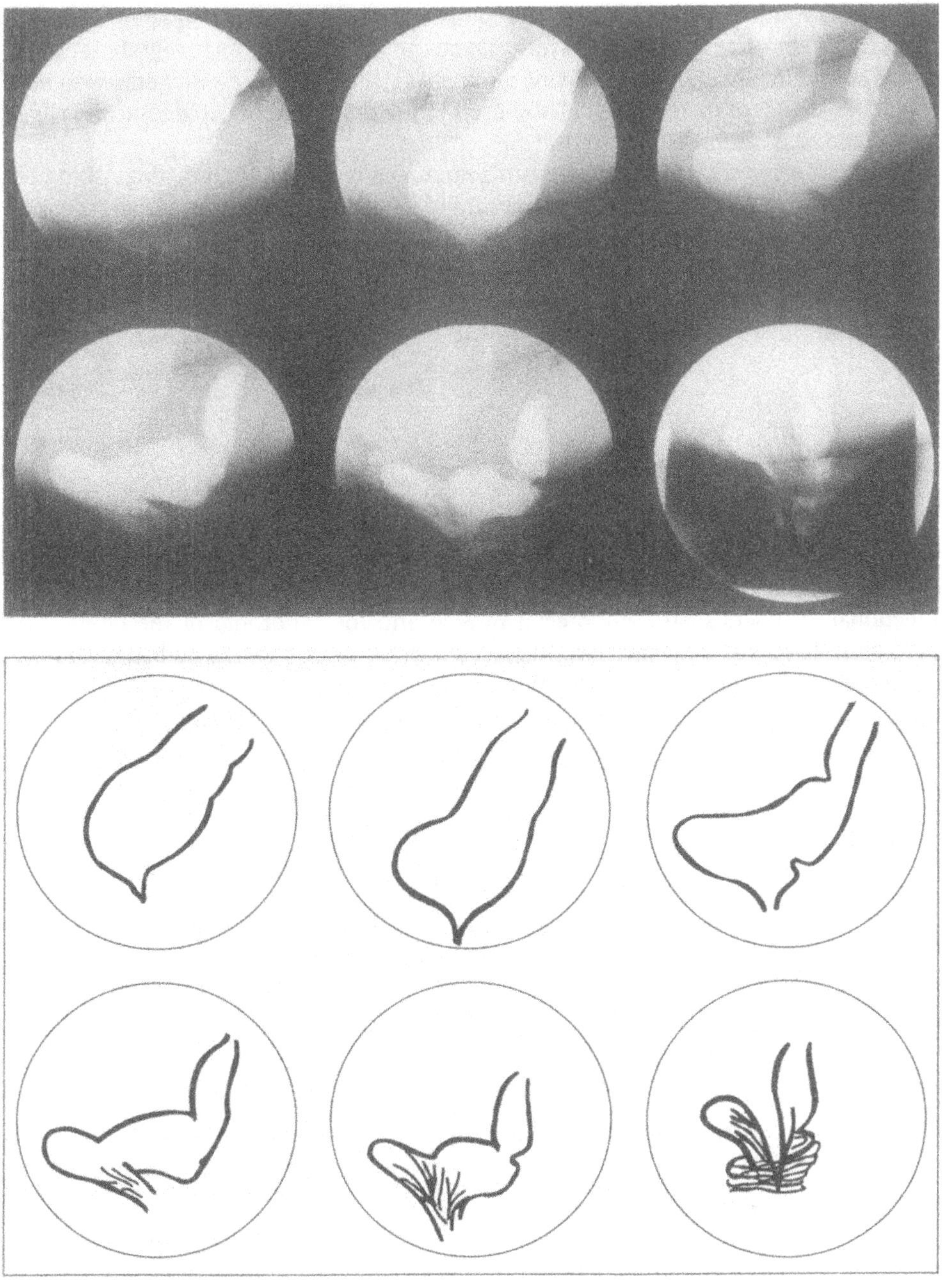

Fig. 6. Association between a rectocele and an intra-anal rectal intussusception

prolapse; a routine procedure which requires no special technical equipment or preliminary colonic preparations and which can be carried out in the relatively short time of 10 - 15 min; the possibility of detecting anomalies which do not reveal themselves until after the ejection of the opaque balloon used in the proctography technique and which thus could pass entirely unnoticed.

It must be mentioned that there can sometimes be difficulty in distinguishing between simple rectal intussusceptions and simple mucous prolapses - especially those intussusceptions which appear in the region beyond the anterior rectal lining. It is possible to base the differential diagnosis on the inversion of the curvature of the anterior lining in the case of an intussusception. This indicates that the whole rectal lining is involved, while in simple mucous prolapse only an incomplete protrusion is apparent in the rectal lumen.

7 Conclusion

Though the balloon proctography technique can be useful, it seems that defecography is a better and more practical routine investigative procedure - probably even more so in specialized units - for the detection of intussusception and rectal prolapse, rectocele, functional disorders of the puborectal muscle and the syndrome of the descending perineum. It allows the clinician to make a choice between medical and surgical treatment and can also play a role in the monitoring of the surgical treatment used for these anomalies (*rectopexy*) and in the long-term evaluation of their efficacy.

References

Bartram Cl, Mahieu P (1985) Radiology of the pelvic floor. In: Henry M. Swash M (eds) Proctology and the pelvic floor, chap 9. Butterworths, London, pp 151 - 186

Broden B, Snellman B (1968) Procidentia of the rectum studied with cineradiography: a contribution to the discussion of causative mechanism. Dis Colon Rectum 11: 330 - 347

Brown B (1965) Defecography or anorectal studies in children including cinefluorographic observation. J Can Assoc Radiol 16: 66 - 76

Burhenne HJ (1964) Intestinal evacuation study: a new roentgenologic technique. Radiol Clin (Basel) 33: 79 - 84

Hardcastle JD, Parks AG (1970) A study of anal incontinence and some principles of surgical treatment. Proc R Soc Med 63: 116 - 118

Kerremans R (1969) Morphological and physiological aspects of anal continence and defecation. Arscia, Brussels

Mahieu P (1983) La Défécographie. Description d'une technique simplifiée et apport diagnostique. Ann Gastroentérol Hépatol (Paris) 19: 345 - 350

Mahieu PHG (1986) Barium enema and defaecography in the diagnosis and evaluation of the solitary ulcer syndrome. Int J Colorect Dis 1: 85 - 90

Mahieu PHG (1987) Defecography in ano-rectal defecation disorders. In: Cola B, Morganti I (eds) Advances in coloproctology. Monduzzi, Bologna, pp 743 - 747

Mahieu P, Pringot J, Vanheuverzwyn R, Goncette L (1981) Les prolapsus du rectum: apport du lavement baryté et de la défécographie. Acta Gastroenterol Belg 44: 501 - 512

Mahieu P, Pringot J, Bodart P (1984a) Defecography: I. Description of a new procedure and results in normal patients. Gastrointest Radiol 9: 247 - 251

Mahieu P, Pringot J, Bodart P (1984b) Defecography: II. Contribution to the diagnosis of defecation disorders. Gastrointest Radiol 9: 253 - 261

Parks AG, Porter NH, Hardcastle JD (1966) The syndrome of the descending perineum. Proc R Soc Med 59: 477 - 482

Phillips SF, Edwards DAW (1965) Some aspects of anal continence and defecation. Gut 6: 396 - 405

Preston DM, Lennard-Jones JE, Thomas BM (1982) The balloon proctogram. Br J Surg 71: 29 - 32

Rutter KPR, Riddell RH (1975) The solitary ulcer syndrome of the rectum. Clin Gastroenterol 4: 505 - 530

Frontiers in European Radiology

Editors-in-Chief:
A. L. Baert, E. Boijsen, W. A. Fuchs, F. Heuck

Springer-Verlag Berlin Heidelberg New York London Paris Tokyo Hong Kong

Volume 1

1982. 113 figures in 187 separate illustrations.
V, 170 pages. Hard cover. ISBN 3-540-10753-3

Volume 2

1982. 70 figures in 84 separate illustrations.
V, 103 pages. Hard cover. ISBN 3-540-11349-5

Contents: *W. Loeffler:* NMR as an Imaging Method. - *R. E. Steiner, G. M. Bydder:* Initial Clinical Experience with NMR Imaging. - *F. W. Smith:* NMR Imaging of the Liver and Kidney. - *P. Marhoff, M. Pfeiler:* Digital Fluorography. - *M. P. Capp, S. Nudelmann, D. Fisher, T. W. Ovitt, G. D. Pond, M. M. Frost, H. Roehrig, J. Seeger, D. Oimette:* Digital Radiography. - *A. B. Crummy, C. A. Mistretta:* Digital Subtraction Arteriography (DSA). - *T. F. Meany, M. A. Weinstein, E. Buonocore, J. H. Gallagher:* Digital Subtraction Angiography: Cleveland Clinic Experience.

Volume 3

1984. 80 figures in 143 separate illustrations.
III, 136 pages. Hard cover. ISBN 3-540-11446-7

Contents: *C. Muhr, K. Bergström:* Modern Evaluation of the Sella Turcica. - *E. Starck, P. Harth, J. Kollath, H. Riemann, S. Tuengerthal, M. Walter:* Clinical Experience with Digital Subtraction Angiography. - *D. Claus:* Brain Ultrasonography in the Infant: A Review. - *P. Suetens, A. Baert, J. Gybels, S. Haegemans, P. Jansen, K. Oosterlinck, G. Wilms:* An Integrated 3-D Image of Cerebral Blood Vessels and CT View of Tumor. - *W. S. Rau, G. Renz, A. Tassinari-Renz, H. Friedburg, U. N. Riede, W. Wenz:* Pulmonary Edema and Shock Lung: Roentgenographic Observations on Pathologic Fine Structure of the Lung.

Springer

Frontiers in European Radiology

Editors-in-Chief:
A. L. Baert, E. Boijsen, W. A. Fuchs, F. Heuck

Volume 4

1984. 82 figures in 144 separate illustrations. I, 158 pages. Hard cover. ISBN 3-540-13410-7

Contents: *P. Lasjaunias, P. Halim, L. Lopez-Ibor:* Therapeutic Angiography in Neuroradiology: Clinical Objectives and Results. – *U. Reiser, J. Buck, F. Heuck:* Densitometric Investigations of Renal Perfusion by Dynamic X-Ray Computed Tomography. – *R. Köster:* Percutaneous Transhepatic Drainage: Technique, Results, and Special Applications. – *H. Fröhlich:* Videodensitometric Measurements of the Blood Flow in the Model Circulation and in the Iliac Arteries: Methodological Investigations.

Volume 5

1987. 120 figures, 33 tables. III, 176 pages. Hard cover. ISBN 3-540-17636-5

Contents: *J. Buck:* Angiocinedensitometry of Renal Blood Circulation by Electrocardiogram-Controlled Injection and Computer Assisted Evaluation. – *C. L. Zollikofer:* Experimental Basis of Percutaneous Transluminal Angioplasty. – *J. Pirschel:* Ultrasound Examination of the Breast. – Diagnostic Information Related to Mammography. – *D. Poos, P. Capesius:* Computerized Tomography in Pituitary Microadenoma.

Springer-Verlag Berlin Heidelberg New York London Paris Tokyo Hong Kong

Springer

GPSR Compliance
The European Union's (EU) General Product Safety Regulation (GPSR) is a set of rules that requires consumer products to be safe and our obligations to ensure this.

If you have any concerns about our products, you can contact us on

ProductSafety@springernature.com

In case Publisher is established outside the EU, the EU authorized representative is:

Springer Nature Customer Service Center GmbH
Europaplatz 3
69115 Heidelberg, Germany

www.ingramcontent.com/pod-product-compliance
Lightning Source LLC
Chambersburg PA
CBHW061223240926
51846CB00006B/1331
* 9 7 8 3 6 4 2 7 4 2 3 5 4 *